# PREGNANCY

## GUIDE FOR FIRST TIME MOMS

The Complete Guide Pregnancy, Childbirth, and the Newborn, What to Expect With Childbirth and Motherhood

**Maria Sunni**

## TABLE OF CONTENTS

# INTRODUCTION

First off, I would like to thank you for choosing this book. I hope that you find the information within these pages helpful and informative so that it can guide you along your pregnancy journey. I know this can be a scary and exciting time, but with the right information, your pregnancy can be a lot easier.

The first thing we will discuss is figuring out if you are ready to be pregnant. This is extremely important and will make all the difference during your pregnancy and motherhood. It will also discuss the process of getting pregnant.

Then we will look at finding out your pregnant. While you won't know for sure until you take a pregnancy test or go to the doctor, there are some early warning signs of pregnancy. Knowing those can help you figure out if you should get the doctors to get tested.

After that, we'll talk about how to get ready for the baby. Babies require a lot of stuff, and it's a good idea to start gathering up those things during pregnancy. However, there may be some things that can wait until later on.

Next, we'll talk about exercise and diet for pregnant women. This can help keep the mom-to-be healthy during pregnancy to make sure her body is ready for labor and care for the growing baby.

Then we will go over what you can expect in each month of pregnancy. This will be broken down into each trimester. Big changes happen to the baby and your body during each trimester, and it's helpful to know what to expect.

After that, we will discuss labor. This is the exciting and scariest part of pregnancy, but there are classes most women take before they give birth to help them prepare. We'll discuss vaginal delivery, as well as C-section. Well, look at what to expect if you have multiple births and how that can look different from single births.

Then we'll talk about the process of bringing baby home. This is something that you will start working on before you ever go into labor. Hopefully, you are ready when the big day arrives.

Next, we'll talk about breastfeeding. If at all possible, breastfeeding is something that all moms should do because it is good for the baby. We'll look at the different aspects of breastfeeding and how to make sure your baby is getting plenty to eat.

After that, we'll go over some health concerns you may need to watch out for so that they don't cause significant problems. These could be baby health problems or health problems in yourself. You never know what can happen, but everything can be treated

Lastly, we will go over ten important points about pregnancy that all new moms should know about.

Before we begin, I would like to ask if you find any part of this book helpful, please leave a review.

# CHAPTER 1: THE JOURNEY OF MATERNITY

You have numerous ovulation kits in your medicine cabinet. You have already picked out your favorite baby names, and you got all of your sister's maternity clothes packed away for when you might need them. How can you know that you are ready to become a mother? I got together with some "mom" friends and acquaintances and asked them to tell me their stories of how they realized they were ready to be a mom.

## How to Know You Are Ready for a Baby

I get asked a lot how I knew I was ready to have a baby. I knew from a young age that I wanted to have children. I loved playing with dolls. I babysat all the neighborhood children and had to smile at all the babies and children I got near. After I met my husband, I knew for sure I was ready to have a baby.

None of our acquaintances had children, but I ached to have a baby in my arms. It was a shocking, visceral, and physical feeling. I talked it over with my soon to be husband, and we agreed we were ready to start trying for a baby. About a month after we returned from the trip, I realized I was pregnant.

Even though I wanted to have children, I was amazed by how motherhood changed my life. We faced all the ups and downs that came along with children. I loved being a parent, but later on, in my life, I finally realized what a colossal decision being a mom really was.

### Young Beginnings

I knew I wanted to be a mother at a young age. My mother didn't have me until she was 34, and she died at the age of 52. I was only 13 years old when she died. I realized that if she had decided to have me when she was younger, we would have had more time together. I wanted to make sure that my children had all the time in the world with me. I had my first child when I was only 23. At the age of 25, I gave birth to twins. I had gotten to be a young mother. I hope that my children will still want me around once I am 98.

### Accidental Baby

My daughter was a complete surprise. We refer to her as the juice cleanse baby. I was using a diaphragm as my birth control. I did my first cleanse when they were popular several years ago. I lost 12 pounds, but I was not aware that weight loss could affect the way a diaphragm fits. Well, it does. I didn't have time to decide if I was ready to have a child; I did have my problems being a mother. I love my daughter, and the experience of being a mom has humbled me, but I didn't have time to become emotionally prepared for the things I had to give up like morning sex, time with my significant other, and alone time. I also didn't know how much willpower and energy it would take to have a career, child, and home life. I didn't understand all the sacrifices I would have to make. It took me a while to find my path.

**A Mormon Experience**

My first child was born when I was 25. It is an everyday occurrence with Mormons to have their children at a young age. Being financially stable wasn't ever a factor. They just assumed that everything would work out. My husband was in law school, and we never even talked about whether we were ready to have children.

My mother gave birth to me when she was young. I was the first of five. My family made sure that they were front and center in the Mormon community. Even though I loved that, how girls were raised was a bit unbalanced. My parents always talked about how excited they were to have me and become a mother. I never once heard them tell me that they couldn't wait to see what I would accomplish with my degree.

They never pressured me. It was an assumption. Females just did it.

I would never want to assume things about my daughter, and I will always say something like: "If you want to be a mom someday, I know you will be a great one." or "If you want to be a doctor someday, I know you will be a great one." I want to make sure that she is raised with a different mindset than I was. I wanted her to know that she had endless possibilities out there and know that there is joy in having choices.

Knowing whether or not I was ready to have children wasn't an option for me. It sounds so silly to admit that. And it does sound a bit foolish. I recently had a friend tell me: "I put so much more thought into which stroller to buy than whether or not to have a child." I am still happy about how things turned out, but it's crazy to think about how things would be for me if I hadn't started having children at such a young age.

### It Was an Intellectual Decision

Since I was the youngest of my siblings, I didn't have to do a lot. I didn't babysit like my older sisters, and I never felt like I needed to have my child. It was just at the back of my mind that once I got married, that urge would appear. So, I continued to wait, and I never got that urge.

Once I reached my mid-30s, my husband and I realized that choosing to have a child would have to be an intelligent choice rather than an emotional one. We were financially stable. We enjoyed staying home on Saturday nights, cuddling on the couch watching Netflix. One of our "couple friends" just got pregnant, and we basically looked at each other and said: "Why not?" I was worried that not having an urge to get pregnant would make it hard for me to "be a mom," but I fell in love with my son when he was born, and I didn't regret my decision. While I will continue to say that I was not ready to become a mom, but I made myself ready.

**There Isn't a Perfect Time**

We knew that we wanted to have children, and since we were nearing our 30s, my husband said that we should get things started. I replied with: "But things are so good the way they are." He disputed with: "There isn't a perfect time to have a baby." He was right.

We had always had some life or career reasons why the time wasn't right, but I understand now that we would have always said it wasn't the right time. I don't believe that anybody has an alarm clock that goes off, telling them that, "Today is the day."

Once our children were born, we had room for them. That's how it works. In my opinion, humans naturally worry about change, but we will adapt and change into something that we never could imagine.

**Long-Term Vision**

My significant other and I sat down one night and talked about what we wanted in our lives in ten, 15, or 20 years. We were trying to decide on something based on a vision. We both wanted to live in a multi-generational, bustling community that had both children and adults in it. We wanted to go to baseball, soccer, and football games and see our children graduate. I was never really, "am I ready to be deprived of sleep?" or "will I find motherhood awesome?" It was more of, "The life we wanted to have when we turned 50, ideally, would have children in it."

I honestly think we just say that we are ready, we will adjust to having children in our life more naturally and efficiently, and we won't ever regret it. If this is true, then nobody will ever be ready. It makes sense to feel unsure about the change in life, and having a bit of ambivalence does not mane that you don't want to or aren't ready to have children.

It is a significant decision to make. It's not liking choosing to go to college, and knowing that if it isn't a good fit for you, you can quit. After you have a child, you will have them for the rest of your life. I think this question is more about trying to figure out if you are going to regret something. If you have children, will you regret it eventually? Will you regret it if you don't have a child? For the majority of people, the answer to both is going to be yes. There are no quizzes out there that will help you not feel nostalgic about the road you chose not to take.

## Only One Child

When I was working at *Elle Magazine*, I overheard a lot of my coworkers talking about the rollercoaster rid of parenthood. I always thought about it. I was never really sure if I would like to be a mom. I also did not know if I didn't want to be a mom. I was at a 50/50 standpoint, totally unsure. My thing was I wanted to be 100 percent before I got into it. I had to want it.

I interviewed a fertility expert, and they told me that you didn't want to get to a point where you wanted a child more than you wanted anything else. Women who get to this point do so because they have tried to have a baby and can't. A different doctor during a different interview suggested that rather than making a "yes" or "no" decision on children, it would be better to think either "just one child" or "more than one child." They pointed out that one child would give you the joy of being a parent without it getting intense with having multiple children. The majority of things that I worried about the most might get affected with just one child, like my finances, relationships, and career.

This was the first time somebody suggested having one child, so we decided to have a child.

Now I have a hard time telling others what it feels like to be a mom. Before I became a mom, it annoyed me when people say, "Once you have a baby, you will love them so much." I would just roll my eyes. Now I struggle with that because it is a great thing. How would I say that to others without coming off as brain-washed and was utterly fascinated with my child? It was completely awesome. Every day I felt 100 percent happy with having my child. This is why I make sure I don't write or talk about being a mother using a tone of "living happily ever after" because it comes off so cliché. I am happy we decided to have a baby.

### A Full Calendar

After I got married, we sat down to find a quiet time in our busy schedules. We waited a few months after our wedding before we took our Italian honeymoon. I knew I wanted to enjoy all the cured meats, cheese, and wines. In the busy year to come, there seemed to be endless life circumstances that always intervened. We were at five weddings. We decided to move. I changed jobs. It went on and on, making our lives more uncertain and hectic.

We thought it made sense to wait until our lives had settled down a bit, and all the weddings and trips were over. I would end up becoming pregnant after the wedding of my best friend. She got pregnant the same month.

## Fingers Crossed Each Month

I was positive I didn't want children during my 20s. I knew without a doubt that I wouldn't want a tiny human that needed me. I loved children, but I also liked having my freedom, so the idea of children wasn't all that important.

Then there was this shift when I turned 32. It wasn't like I was struck by lightning; it was more of a slow change. I took some time to get my cycles in sync. I worked on my general fertility for some time. I read the book *Women's Bodies, Women's Wisdom*. I changed up the way that I cared for myself and what I ate.

I began welcoming the idea of having a child. I began talking about it with my boyfriend. I started feeling emotionally connected with the idea of having a family. We weren't wondering about it; we were hoping for it.

When I turned 35, we hoped each month that we would get pregnant. The journey was long, and it took us a lot of turns and twists, but we finally figured out we were pregnant right before I turned 39. I am 30 weeks along, and we aren't at the end of our story just yet. I feel grateful for where I am, and I am always going to respect and remember how long this process took.

The best advice I can give you about "figuring out if you are ready" just takes you time. There are too many people who run around but do the same things with huge decisions in life. People say that our lives move fast, but I don't see it this way. If we just pay attention, our lives will move more slowly. There is a lot out there for us to learn from each day. If you start to pay attention to your life, you will figure out when you are ready, and if this pondering over it ends up being part of the journey, there isn't anything wrong with that. I hope everyone has a wonderful path on their journey to motherhood.

If the above stories didn't help you figure out if you are ready to have a baby, some signs might help you know. Well, you know if the internet gives you a list that shows you are prepared for a baby, then you are absolutely ready.

- You've Seen Other People With Their Children and You Think You Can Be Better

You see a mom at the park, and you decide to judge her because her children have ice cream of the hands and face. Her children might be sitting quietly eating their ice cream, and she decides to check her messages, and you automatically say she's an unobservant mom. Your self-righteousness and optimism are just adorable. You are going to be that mom one day, and some childless "holier-than-thou know-it-all" is going to judge you. This is the circle of being a parent.

- You Have Seen An Episode of *A Baby Story*

There will be a brief time in your life when this show will appeal to you. It is the peach schnapps of the television world. If you can watch an entire episode, you are ready to have a baby. If you recorded an episode to watch later, take a pregnancy test now.

- None of Your Furnishings Are White

At one time, I had a white sofa, and then this cute, small person drew on it with a blue marker. If you love your white things, you aren't ready for children. These two things are mutually exclusive. Most parents will have brown things for a good reason, and it isn't because it looks nice. It is because it hides stains, spills, etc.

- You Love The Night Life and Morning Life

You sit up to watch Jimmy Kimmel, but you are up early enough to see the sun come up each morning. You aren't going to miss anything.

- You Can Wash Your Clothes In A Washing Machine

Either that or your family owns a dry-cleaning business. These are your only two options.

- You Eat Your Friends Leftovers and Crusts

This will be about 40 percent of your meals after you have a child. It is a good idea to eat it now to see if you can handle it. You get bonus points if you have picked crumbs off a person's shirt and eaten them without thinking.

- You Feel Well-Rested

The one thing that you will constantly hear when you get pregnant is, "bank your sleep now." Once you get pregnant, you will not get enough sleep because you will be peeing once every hour and getting kicked in the ribs by a fetus that refuses to sleep when you are ready to sleep. Basically, you have to get all your sleeping done before you get pregnant.

- You Love Looking At Babies

You don't look at them like "I hope that baby isn't on my flight." You look at them in "look at those chubby little hands" kind of way.

- You Don't Mind Bodily Fluids

Your child is going to leak everything all over the place. At times it might be everything at one time, and it will get all over you. I can't count the number of times my daughter pooped on me.

- You Love To Share

You better prepare yourself to never finish anything by yourself again.

- You Love Showing Off Your Breasts

They look the best right now than they are ever going to look. Now is when you should be showing them off. They may get a lot bigger while you are pregnant and nursing, but the veins in them will get prominent, too. Did nobody bother telling you this? Sorry, surprise. They are also going to deflate like sad balloons. If you do decide to breastfeed, there will be fewer people in your social circle who haven't seem your boobs than the people who have. Maybe you should take a picture of them now just in case you want to show someone what they used to be like.

- You Love Drinking By Yourself

Do you know those days when you just wanted to unwind by drinking a glass or two of wine with some friends? Well, it is going to be hard to meet up with them when you are a tiny human's milking machine, or you are waking up every three to four hours. If you consume wine in moderation and safely a couple of hours before you will nurse again, they will love you forever.

- You Witnessed a Temper Tantrum and Didn't Run For The Hills

Each time my child would have a temper tantrum, I felt like Trojan owed me money for free advertising. If you have seen a temper tantrum, and you still feel like you want to procreate, this is a good sign. If you feel relaxed because you think your "perfect little angel" won't have temper tantrums, you are so wrong.

- You Love Television and Going Out

Eventually, you will get to go out again, but if you are a new, sleep-deprived parent, you are going to use all your free time to get caught up on sleep, eating, and maybe once a week, you get a shower. Here are some things you can do: watch any show where the characters actually get to leave their house. This will be the same thing, except your version won't have to worry about getting dressed up, meeting your friends, or drinking and eating great tasting foods.

- You Get Pregnant

Don't let anything you read above scare you away. You are going to be awesome.

**How to Have a Healthy Pregnancy**

If you have decided that you are ready to have a baby, here are some ways to get your pregnancy off to a good start. These things can be done before you start trying to get pregnant to help your fertility and how healthy your baby and pregnancy are.

- Be Ready

About one in every three women will get pregnant in the first month they try to get pregnant, so you need to be ready for your pregnancy. How healthy you are before you get pregnant will set the foundation for your baby's health. If you can follow the advice below, you will be able to:

  - Reduce the risk of developing complications during pregnancy
  - Improves your fertility
  - Protect the development of your baby and its future health

When you begin trying to get pregnant, you aren't going to know that you are pregnant for a few weeks. You need to make some healthy lifestyle changes now instead of waiting because it will give you peace when your pregnancy test comes up positive.

You have to stop:

- Recreational drugs
- Alcohol
- Smoking

The following things will improve your chances of having a healthy baby and pregnancy:

- Get tested for STDs if you think there is a possibility you might have one.
- Make sure you have had the MMR vaccine since rubella can harm a developing baby.
- Have a pap smear if you haven't had one in the past year.
- Stay active or get active as this an improve fertility and can make your baby and pregnancy healthier
- If you are overweight, try to lose some weight.
- Cut down on caffeine if you drink a lot. Go to just one cup a day.
- Eat a balanced diet as it can improve your fertility and affects your baby's health, too.
- Begin taking folic acid now. It takes time to build up in the body.

- Track Your Menstrual Cycle

Some women know the exact date their period will begin, but most won't be sure after taking contraceptives for a long time.

Write down the day your period begins on a calendar. Your complete cycle starts on this day and goes until the next time you begin bleeding. This can give you a good starting point on how long your cycle is and allows you to figure out when you could be ovulating. This is when your egg gets released so it can be fertilized.

There are many pregnancy apps out there that could help you track your cycle and dates you might be ovulating.

If you have recently stopped taking your contraceptives, your periods might get a bit irregular for a couple of months until your body gets used to the hormone level change.

- Never Stop Any Medications Without Consulting Your Doctor

If you are currently taking any medicine for a mental or physical health problem, talk with your doctor about them before you begin trying to get pregnant. NEVER stop taking any medications because your symptoms might come back, or they might get worse. Your doctor will know what will be safest for you and your baby.

- Don't Get Too Anxious

Trying to get pregnant can make you anxious for several reasons. You have to take care of your mental health, just like taking care of your body during pregnancy.

- Know When You Need to Seek Fertility Help

If you haven't gotten pregnant within one year of having regular unprotected sex, you need to talk with your doctor. If you have problems like PCOS, endometriosis, or over 36 years old, speak to your doctor after only six months.

**Getting Pregnant**

If you want to get pregnant, you have to get your eggs and your significant other's sperm together as many times as possible. About eight out of ten couples will get pregnant within one year of having regular unprotected sex as long as they are under that age of 40. About nine out of ten couples will be pregnant in two years.

To have regular unprotected sex means that you will have sex every two to three days with no protection.

There is no need to make sure you only have sex when you're ovulating, even though it does help if you are aware of your ovulation time. Making sure that you have vaginal sex several times a week will help to keep your chances good. Sperm is able to live around three days once in the vagina. That means you are having sex regularly, and then there is a good chance that sperm will be in your vagina when your body releases an egg

Just remember to keep sex enjoyable by concentrating on the relationship and each other instead of worrying about getting pregnant. This is going to help you lessen your stress.

### How Pregnancy Starts

Your cycle begins on the first day you start bleeding and goes until the first day of your next period. You can expect the following to happen during your cycle and the beginning of your pregnancy.

- Eggs get mature in the ovaries each month
- The womb lining will get thicker to get ready for a fertilized egg
- When the egg gets matured, the ovary releases it, and this is when you are ovulating
- During this time, your cervical mucus will get clearer and thinner. This helps the sperm swim to the egg
- When you have sex, millions of sperm swim up and through the cervix, into the uterus and on into the fallopian tubes to meet the egg

- If sperm is there at ovulation, or within 24 hours, the egg might get fertilized. It only takes one sperm
- If the egg gets fertilized, it will begin to move toward the uterus and begin to split
- When it reaches the uterus, the egg needs to attach to the lining of the uterus. This is what is referred to as implantation, and it marks the start of your pregnancy. The majority of fertilized eggs will not implant and simply passes through the body.
- If the egg doesn't get fertilized, the egg gets reabsorbed into the body, your hormone levels will drop, and the lining of the uterus receives shed. You have now started your period.

**When to Have Sex So You Can Get Pregnant**

To boost your chances of getting pregnant, try to have regular sex during your cycle, so you know there is a lot of sperm in the uterus when to egg gets released. Having an active sex life is necessary to get pregnant.

If you already keep track of your cycle and know when your ovulation occurs, you will have a better chance of becoming pregnant when you have sex during the week before and during ovulation. You need to have sex still while you are ovulating. Once this is over, your most fertile time will be done for this cycle.

### Is There a Better Sex Position That Helps You Get Pregnant?

The sex position doesn't matter for conception as long as the man ejaculates inside the vagina. After that, the sperm will start to make their way up through the cervix, through the uterus, and then into the fallopian tubes where it meets the egg.

Some say that a woman can raise her legs up after sex to help the sperm get into the uterus, but no evidence proves this is true. Going from the vagina into the uterus isn't a straight line, so you don't have to worry about the sperm coming back out if you stand up to have sex or after sex.

### When Will You Be Ovulating

Ovulation happens typically around ten to 16 days before the beginning of your period. This is why you need to know the length of your cycle before you begin trying to get pregnant.

There is a chance that you won't know when your ovulation day is, and if you have been taking a contraceptive, there is a good chance that you have had a normal cycle your started taking the pill.

The first thing to do is to mark on a calendar the dates that you bleed. You will be able to count the number of days from the first day to your next period to find the length of your cycle.

You might experience some of these changes that will help you know when you are ovulating:

- Temperature

You can learn more about your menstrual cycle if you start recording your temperature each morning as soon as you get up. The temperature will rise by around 0.2 degrees if ovulation has happened.

Since it only shows you after you have ovulated, and can't tell you when your most fertile days begin, most women don't find it very helpful.

- Changes in Cervical Mucus

A woman's cervix will secrete mucus during the menstrual cycle. In the beginning, it will be sticky white and will gradually get clearer and thinner. Before and then during ovulation, the mucus will increase and gets more stretchy, slippery, and thinner. Women compare it to a raw egg white.

This thin mucus helps the sperm get to the egg easier. On the last day, you notice the thinner mucus; it is known as the "peak day," which happens extremely close to when ovulation occurs.

# CHAPTER 2: HURRAY! YOU THINK YOU'RE PREGNANT

Did you know that there are earlier signs of pregnancy than missing your period? The proof may be in the pregnancy test, but even before you ever miss your period, you could suspect that you are pregnant. Knowing the first signs and why they happen can help you spot pregnancy early on.

## The Classics

There are common signs of pregnancy that most of us are probably already aware of, but let's go over them.

1. Missed Period

We all learned this in school that the first sign you are pregnant is missing your period. If a week or more goes by without the start of an expected menstrual cycle, especially if you are always regular, there is a chance that you might be pregnant. That said, this might not be reliable if you don't have a regular cycle.

2. Swollen, Tender Breasts

All of the hormonal changes taking place during the early part of your pregnancy can cause the breasts to become sore and sensitive. The discomfort will generally decrease after a couple of weeks once your body has gotten used to the hormonal changes. You may also notice that your areolas are becoming darker and bumpy. Estrogen and progesterone should be blamed for this early sign of pregnancy. The pain you will be experiencing, though, is getting everything ready for the milk-making that will happen later on.

The areolas can also increase in size. You may notice you have tiny bumps growing in size and numbers on your areola as well. These bumps are known as Montgomery's tubercles. They were always there, but they are getting ready to produce more oils to lubricate your nipples once the baby begins to nurse.

You can help relieve some of the pain and tenderness by wearing a supportive and comfortable maternity bra. Often, the most comfortable ones will be cotton and underwire-free. Pick out a bra with varying clasps so that you have more room to "grow" as the baby gets bigger. You can also purchase breast pads that you can place in the bra to reduce friction on the nipples.

3. Nausea With or Without Vomiting

Morning sickness, which can hit at any point during the day, often starts one month after becoming pregnant. However, some women will experience nausea very early on, and some won't ever experience. While the cause of this nausea during pregnancy remains unclear, the hormones are the likely culprit.

If you do experience morning sickness, it's a good idea to keep saltine crackers with you. Keeping a pack next to your bed and eating a few before you get up each morning can settle the morning sickness. Staying hydrated is also important, so make sure you drink plenty of water. Ginger ale can also help settle an upset stomach. If you are unable to keep anything down, contact your doctor.

4. Increased Urination

You might find that you have to pee more often than usual. This can happen two to three weeks after conception. How much blood you have in your body increases when you are pregnant, which causes your kidneys to process more fluid that will end up in your bladder. The pregnancy hormone hCG causes an increase in blood flow to the kidneys. The growing uterus will also add more pressure on your bladder, making less storage space for urine.

5. Fatigue

Imagine hiking up a mountain without training with a heavy backpack that gains a little more weight each day. That's basically what pregnancy is. It's tough, which is why fatigue is prevalent. Fatigue is probably one of the more reliable early symptoms of pregnancy. Generally, all women will experience this because of the levels of progesterone soar, which makes you feel tired. You also use a large amount of energy to build a placenta, which is the life-support for your baby. All of this can end up zapping your usual get-up-and-go and can cause you to feel fatigued shortly after you have conceived.

**Less Common Signs of Pregnancy**

The answer to whether or not you might be pregnant could lie within one of these lesser-known signs of pregnancy. If you don't experience any of these early ones, don't worry, not everybody will.

1. Moodiness

With the flood of pregnancy hormones in your body early in the pregnancy it can make you unusually emotional and weepy. It is prevalent to have mood swings. As early as week four into the pregnancy, you could experience PMS-like moodiness. Later one, and throughout the remainder of your pregnancy, you could find yourself anxious one minute and depressed the next.

Besides all of the hormones coursing through your body right now, your life is getting ready to change in a big way, so it's normal for your mood to go crazy. Do what you can to give yourself a break, eat well, and make sure you are getting plenty of rest.

2. Bloating

The first hormonal changes can cause you to feel bloated, a lot like how you could feel when you start your period. Finding your jeans fitting a little snugger it could be because of this. While you can't blame this puffiness on your baby just yet, you can blame progesterone, which will slow down your digestion, ensure that nutrients from your foods get into the bloodstream and reach the baby.

3. Light Spotting

Some women will have a small amount of light spotting as their first sign of pregnancy. This is what is referred to as implantation bleeding, and occurs once the fertilized egg attaches to the uterus. This typically occurs about ten to 14 days after conception. Implantation bleeding will naturally happen around the time your period was supposed to start. However, not every woman will experience this. Some women will experience mild uterine cramping early on in the pregnancy as well.

During week one to week four, everything is occurring on a cellular level. The fertilized egg has started to make a blastocyst that will start forming into organs and body parts for the baby. At around week four, after the conception, this blastocyst will implant in the endometrium, which is the uterine lining. This is when the implantation bleeding can occur, which a woman may mistake for a light period.

4. Constipation

Changes in hormones can cause the digestive system to slow down, which can end up causing constipation.

5. Food Aversions

When you are pregnant, you could find that you are more sensitive to certain smells, and you may have a change in your sense of taste. You could see one of your favorite foods, and you could find that it is causing your stomach to turn, or it could contribute to morning sickness. Chicken is a very common food aversion, but it can be as odd as a salad. This likely because of a heightened sense of smell. This causes even mild odors unappealing and strong. If you find your sniffer is easily offended, you could be pregnant. Like a lot of other symptoms of pregnancy, these food preferences can be caused by hormonal changes.

Food aversion doesn't tend to show up super early on in a pregnancy, but it will typically occur during the first three months. Don't worry; this will pass by the second trimester when all of the hormones have settled down.

6. Nasal Congestion

With the increase in blood production and hormone levels can cause your mucous membranes in your nose to swell, dry out, and bleed easily. This could cause you to have a runny or stuffy nose.

7. Raised Basal Body Temperature

If you have been taking your basal temperature to help get pregnant, you may notice that it rises about a degree once you have conceived and will stay elevated throughout your entire pregnancy. While this is not a sure sign of pregnancy, there are other reasons for a rise in body temperature; it could give you some advance notice.

8. Increased Heart Rate

Around weeks eight and ten, your heart will likely start to pump faster and harder. Arrhythmias and palpitations are common occurrences during pregnancy, and they are perfectly normal because of the hormonal changes. Normally, this is harmless, but if you have underlying heart problems, make sure you are under a doctor's supervision and receive proper medication.

Most of the time, blood pressure will drop during the early stages of pregnancy. This can cause you to feel dizzy since the blood vessels are dilated. There are cases where women experience high blood pressure due to their pregnancy, but that is hard to determine. Nearly all cases of hypertension during the first 20 weeks of pregnancy indicate that there was an underlying problem, to begin with. This problem may not have been present beforehand, but developed during pregnancy. Your doctor will take a blood pressure reading during your first visit to get a baseline for your normal blood pressure.

Unfortunately, a lot of these symptoms of pregnancy are not unique to pregnancy. Some of them could indicate that you are getting sick or getting ready to start your period. Likewise, you could be pregnant without ever experiencing any of these symptoms. Still, if you do miss your period and you have a couple of the other signs, take a pregnancy test or pay a visit to your doctor. The sooner you know you are pregnant, the sooner you can start your prenatal care.

**How Soon Can Pregnancy Signs Appear?**

The very early signs of pregnancy, such as tender breasts and sensitivity to smell, could show up before you ever miss a period, possibly as soon as a couple of days after conception. Other signs, like spotting, may appear about a week after conception. Others, like urinary frequency, will normally show up about two weeks or so after conception.

That said, early signs of pregnancy can show up at various times for different women. Some experience very few, if any, of these symptoms until a month or more into their pregnancy. While some don't experience any of the symptoms, others will suffer from them all. If you have skipped a period, are feeling tired, nauseous, spotting, and have tender beasts, then you may want to drop by a drug store to pick up an at-home pregnancy test, and then on to the doctor to confirm it.

While it may sound odd, the first week of pregnancy is determined from your last menstrual period. The last time you had your period is counted as week one of your pregnancy, even if you weren't pregnant at that time. The first day of your pregnancy is the first day of the last period you had. This is why during those first few weeks, you didn't have any symptoms, but it still counts towards the 40 weeks. To give you an idea of when symptoms typically show up, here is an estimated timeline from your missed period.

- Mild cramping and spotting - week one to four
- Missed period - week four
- Fatigue - week four or five
- Nausea - week four to six
- Aching breasts or tingling - week four to six
- Frequent urination - week four to six
- Bloating - week four to six
- Motion sickness - week five to six
- Mood swings - week six
- Temperature changes - week six
- High blood pressure - week eight
- Extreme fatigue and heartburn - week nine
- Faster heartbeat - week eight to ten
- Breast and nipple changes - week 11
- Acne - week 11
- Noticeable weight gain - week 11
- Pregnancy glow - week 12

**When Can I Take a Test?**

If you are experiencing any of those pregnancy symptoms, you may want to go out and buy a test right away, but it's important to understand what is happening to know the appropriate time to take a test.

After an egg is fertilized, it will travel into the uterus and implant into the uterine wall. During this time, there are tiny amounts of the pregnancy hormone, hCG, that starts to appear in your urine. This is the hormone that all pregnancy tests are made to detect. Some pregnancy tests are made to pick up on pregnancy earlier than others, such as Clearblue Early Detection. They say they can tell six days sooner than your missed period. Even if you take an early detection test, and it shows that you aren't pregnant, you could still be pregnant. The reason for this is that the levels of hCG in women can vary from woman to woman, and you may not have enough of the hormone in your urine for the test to give you a positive result. These hormone levels rise rapidly early on, which means you could take another test on your expected period data, and your result could change.

Most professionals will tell you to wait until the week after your missed period. It will give you the most accurate results. If you want to take a test before you miss your period, at least wait a couple of weeks after you have had sex. Remember, your body needs to develop detectable levels of hCG. This can take anywhere from seven to 12 days after the egg has been successfully implanted.

### When Should I Go to the Doctor?

Most of the time, women will take a home pregnancy test first to determine whether or not they should get to the doctor. If the home pregnancy test is positive, schedule an appointment with you OB/GYN as soon as possible. Doctors have a more sensitive test, such as blood tests and a pelvic exam, that will make sure you are indeed pregnant.

Every pregnancy test, whether ClearBlue, First Response, EPT, or at a doctor's office, work by detecting hCG in the urine. The difference between a urine pregnancy test at the doctor's office versus at home is not within the test but within the interpreter of the test.

There are two tests that doctors can do as well. They can do a urine and blood test–both tests for hCG. The first thing a doctor will do is a urine test in their office. After the urine is tested, the doctor may also do a blood test and a sonogram.

The blood test is done less often than urine tests. Blood tests can detect pregnancy much earlier than a home test. It will take longer to get the results of the blood test, typically two to three days, whereas the urine test results will be available the same day. Most doctor's offices don't have the equipment for blood analysis.

There are two types of blood tests. One is qualitative, and it tests for the presence of hCG in the blood and will give a yes or no. Doctors will normally order these tests to confirm pregnancy earlier on in the pregnancy. They are seldom used to confirm pregnancy quickly.

The second is a quantitative blood test. This measures the exact amounts of hCG that is in your blood. It can discover some of the lowest levels of hCG. Since measures the concentration of hCG, it can be helpful to use to track any issues that might arise during pregnancy. Quantitative tests are generally done to rule out an ectopic pregnancy or to monitor for a miscarriage when the levels tend to fall rapidly.

The doctor will also do a sonogram after they have done a urine test. This uses reflected sound waves to create a picture of the fetus. Sonograms can be used to determine the gestational age of the fetus. This can let you know about how far along you are in your pregnancy. It can also find out if you are having more than one. A transvaginal sonogram is typically done early one to figure out the fetal age or to detect a possible ectopic pregnancy.

For a transvaginal sonogram, you will have to go in with a full bladder. The vaginal transducer, which looks like a wand, is covered with a condom or latex sleeve and vaginal lubricant. You will like back with your hips tilted up slightly. The transducer is gently inserted into the vagina, and the doctor will rotate and move it around to adjust the view on the monitor. There is typically no discomfort. There are no known risks, either.

While nobody wants to think about it, there is a chance that you could have an ectopic pregnancy. Under normal conditions, the egg will attach itself to the uterus. With an ectopic pregnancy, the fertilized egg was unable to move out of the fallopian tubes and will implant in the fallopian tube.

An ectopic pregnancy is not able to grow the way it should, and the egg won't be able to survive. The growing tissue could destroy various structures. If undetected, the egg will grow and eventually bursts into the fallopian tube, which will cause hemorrhaging. If it is left untreated, severe blood loss can result in death. Early treatment can preserve the woman's life and help their chances of future healthy pregnancies.

An ectopic pregnancy may not give any indication of pregnancy. Some signs could be a missed period, nausea, breast tenderness, fatigue, and vomiting. A pregnancy test will show up as positive. But it is not viable. The first signs that it is ectopic includes:

- Cramping on one side of the pelvis
- Lower abdominal pain
- Light vaginal bleeding

If you experience a ruptured fallopian tube, you experience:

- Lightheadedness
- Dizziness
- Sharp, stabbing pains in the abdomen, pelvis, and possibly the neck and shoulder

Most often, an ectopic pregnancy occurs if the fallopian tube is misshapen, scarred, or damaged. Sometimes the cause is just a mystery. Ectopic pregnancies only account for one to two percent of all pregnancies.

# CHAPTER 3: PREPARING FOR PREGNANCY

◆◇◆

Planning for pregnancy starts way before conception for a lot of women. Other women won't begin planning until they know they are pregnant. Even though it's possible to have a healthy baby and pregnancy without planning, creating a pregnancy plan is a way to help make sure your baby has the best chance of being healthy and that your pregnancy will be healthy. Pregnancy planning normally involves the following:

Talking with your partner and health care professionals includes talking about exercise, vitamins, nutrition, genetic counseling, and weight gain. Plus making sure you stay away from alcohol and specific medicines.

You might have to plan for fertility by scheduling time to have sex when you are most fertile. If you are having regular sex, and you don't conceive within one year of having unprotected sex, you might want to begin talking with a fertility expert. If you are over 35, you might want to talk to a fertility expert after six months of trying to get pregnant.

Since implantation bleeding occurs in some women, it may coincide when their period starts, so they may not realize they are pregnant until other symptoms show up. This is true for women who have irregular cycles. By this time, she might have exposed herself to harmful substances without knowing it. Women who choose to start planning for their pregnancy before they get pregnant can take all necessary steps to avoid any possible exposures to harmful substances.

## Why Is Pregnancy Planning Important?

Before you get pregnant, you can talk about your medical history with your doctor but make sure you focus on all the following:

If you have any chronic medical conditions such as heart disease, kidney disease, thyroid disease, or diabetes, your doctor will need to monitor all of these and make sure they are under control before you get pregnant to give you the best chances of having a healthy pregnancy.

You might want to be tested to make sure you haven't been infected with hepatitis B or HIV so that the right treatments can be given during pregnancy or at birth. This can prevent transmitting infections to the baby.

Your doctor will need to know your immunization history and your immune response to rubella and varicella. A simple blood test can figure out your immunity to these infections that could harm the developing fetus. If you aren't immune to these infections, your doctor can give you a vaccine for them before you get pregnant. After you get the varicella vaccine, you will need to wait for one month before you try to conceive. Precautions against developing specific infections need to be taken, too.

If either you or your partner has a history of diseases that have been inherited, have children who have a genetic disease, or have a family history of specific conditions, might decide to undergo some genetic counseling before conceiving. Your doctor can help you decide if you need to have genetic counseling.

If you can stop smoking before conceiving, it can drastically improve your chances of having a healthy pregnancy. Women who are planning their pregnancy should stop drinking alcohol, too. Any type of substance abuse needs to be identified and treated before you plan on getting pregnant.

## How Much Weight Will You Gain?

Your pre-pregnancy weight needs to be considered when trying to estimate the amount of weight you should gain to have a healthy pregnancy. Women who are pregnant with twins, triplets, etc. will need to gain more weight than a woman who is just carrying one fetus. Your doctor can help you determine what is right for you.

## Drinking Alcohol While Pregnant

FASDs or Fetal alcohol spectrum disorders are a group of problems that show the possible effects of the fetus being exposed to alcohol. These could include ARND or alcohol-related neurodevelopmental disabilities, ARBD or alcohol-related birth defects, or FAS or fetal alcohol syndrome. FAS is one of the leading causes of cognitive disabilities. Researchers and doctors have yet to figure out the exact amount of alcohol that an expectant mother would have to ingest to cause FAS, so that's why there is no safe amount of alcohol a mother can consume during her pregnancy. Because of this, women who are planning on getting pregnant and women who are already pregnant needs to stop drinking immediately.

## Having Sex While Pregnant

Having sex during pregnancy is usually safe for most women. Your doctor could recommend avoiding sex if you have specific risk factors or conditions. These might include placenta previa, amniotic fluid leak, bleeding, infection, multiple miscarriages, and preterm labor. Women who are pregnant shouldn't have sex that will put them at risk for contracting an STD.

## Can a Pregnant Woman Fly?

Occasionally traveling by air is safe during pregnancy. There isn't any data that shows air travel will have any adverse effects on the outcome of pregnancy for women who travel occasionally. Most airlines will let a pregnant woman fly up to their 36th week. Those who have been told their pregnancy is high-risk, those who are at a greater risk for preterm labor, or who might need emergency care, should avoid air travel. Women who do choose to travel by air need to make sure that they take the proper precautions to lower their risk of developing blood clots in their feet and legs. Wearing support socks, walking around often, and staying hydrated can reduce the risk of getting blood clots in their legs on long flights.

### Parvovirus B19 and Genital Herpes

Parvovirus B19 can cause fifth disease. This is a common childhood disease that gets spread by blood or respiratory secretions. Pregnant women who haven't had fifth disease need to stay away from anyone who has these conditions because parvovirus B19 can infect the fetus. If a woman develops parvovirus B19 during pregnancy can transmit the infection across the placenta and to the fetus. Even though there haven't been any congenital disabilities reported because of fifth disease, this infection could cause the fetus to die. If a woman contracts this disease during the first trimester, the rate of fetal death could be about ten percent. Staying away from people who have fifth disease could reduce the chances of being infected.

If a woman who is pregnant has genital herpes, there is a possibility to transmit the virus to the baby at birth. Herpes can have many different adverse reactions in a newborn baby. Their infection could be only in the skin, mouth, or eyes. It could also target the central nervous system, or it could be throughout their body. The baby can be given antiviral medications once they are born. Cesarean deliveries are recommended for women who have an active outbreak when they go into labor to keep from spreading the infection to the baby.

**Are You Mentally Ready?**

Guidance about preparing for pregnancy ordinarily centers around all the physical perspectives like taking vitamins, eating right, and exercising to prepare your body. Yet, shouldn't something be said about being mentally ready for being pregnant? Are there things you can do before you get pregnant to ensure your mental wellbeing stays flawless during the pregnancy? Are there any methodologies you can never really limit any intricacies like postpartum depression?

Studies have indicated that mental wellbeing during pregnancy can have impacts on the result of the birth, alongside your psychological states during the baby blues time. Regardless of whether you have a hard pregnancy or if the experience isn't what you figured it would be, there are a few stages you can take to keep you intellectually adjusted.

We should take a look at some ways in which you can get yourself mentally ready.

**Know Your Risks**

Postpartum depression is probably the most serious problem that affects many new mothers. Depression is the main cause of non-obstetric hospitalizations among women. Since PPD could have a huge impact on both the baby and mother's health, so finding ways to keep this from happening and treating the disorder are important.

Are there things you can do to help lower your chances of being bothered by postpartum depression?

Realizing the danger components of PPD could help. While it is unimaginable to expect to foresee who will and won't be influenced, realizing the danger factors you may have will assist you with searching for the principal side effects and signs.

Ladies who have a more serious danger of developing PPD include:

- Women who have a support system that is poor.
- Women who have a history of pregnancy complications or stressful events in life.

- Women who have a family history of postpartum depression
- Women who have conflict in their marriage
- Women who have suffered from PPD before
- Women who already have a history of anxiety and depression

Scientists have found that there are some steps women can take to reduce or prevent PPD. One investigation done in 2015 found that ladies who got mental or psychosocial help were not as prone to encounter misery once they have had a child. The best interventions found in the study include postpartum midwife care, postpartum phone support, postpartum home visits, and interpersonal therapy. Some proof shows that early intellectual conduct treatment could be utilized to forestall post birth anxiety.

Depression after birth could range in severity, but some symptoms you need to look for include:

- Intrusive thoughts
- Anxiety
- Not interested in your baby
- Suicidal thoughts
- Crying
- Feeling inadequate
- Problems concentrating

On the off chance that you think you have PPD manifestations or other concerning emotions, ensure you talk about them with your PCP. Your doctor could recommend treatment like support groups, medications, psychotherapy, self-care, or a combination of these.

When you learn about postpartum depression, its symptoms, and taking note of them gives you the chance to talk to your doctor about what you can do. This can help you at any time during your pregnancy.

## Knowing What to Expect

Getting yourself intellectually ready for your pregnancy implies you need to fabricate a comprehension of what you could envision during your pre-birth period. Pregnancy may incorporate the surprising and the normal. The unexpected may be getting put on bed rest, pica, or sickness. The normal may be pains, aches, peculiar food desires, or weight gain. Before you get pregnant, you have to find out as much about the absolute most basic manifestations that are related to pregnancy, alongside a portion of the more uncommon confusions that you could understanding.

The most significant thing you have to recall is that you could peruse all the magazines, sites, and books that you can discover; however, the startling could occur. You can't anticipate precisely how your pregnancy will go, so you truly need to hold up until you are in it to discover. You simply need to instruct yourself pretty much all the high points and low points.

However, it would be best if you acknowledged that you couldn't control, foresee, or know it all.

**Find Support**

Having solid social help during your pre-birth period is important. This help may originate from your companions, guardians, relatives, or your partner. An examination from 1976 indicated that social help could give you a defensive impact against all the outcomes of worry in your life. Different investigations have discovered that social help during the time paving the way to and afterward after birth affects the mother's emotional wellness.

Besides, social help during your pregnancy can improve the results of birth by bringing down the danger of having an untimely birth. Social help can diminish both pressure and nervousness, alongside enhancing the lady's pressure to deal with stress.

So what are a few things you can do to ensure you have the instructive, passionate, and substantial help that you need previously, during, and after your pregnancy?

- Join an expecting parent's group. It is useful to impart your encounters to different couples who are experiencing very similar things you are. Child rearing, breastfeeding, labor, and pregnancy classes could be some acceptable spots to meet individuals who could offer more help during pregnancy.

- Lean on friends and family. Pregnancy can be hard, especially if your area dealing with some complications like severe morning sickness or other medical problems. Let other people know when you need help.
- Talk with your partner. If you have a spouse or mate who will be an aspect of your kid and your life, take the time and exertion to ensure this relationship is solid. Discussion about any worries and request any assistance when you incline that you need it.

**What You Need for Baby**

There is a lot you have to do when you are getting ready for a baby. Getting all the essentials for baby isn't the least among them. From getting all the sleeping gear, getting the nursery ready, buying diapers, and eating gear, it is easy to say busy just buying all the things your baby has to have. All the things that a newborn baby needs could take any new mom by surprise. How can you figure out which baby items you don't need to worry about and what things you absolutely can't live without? First of all, don't start getting stressed over it. Below you will find a complete breakdown of everything you might possibly need.

**Nursery**

Most women believe that a nursery calls for cute décor, but you are going to need baby bedding and furniture that will make taking care of your baby safer and easier. Here is what is needed for any nursery:

- Bassinet, cradle, or crib
- Three waterproof mattress covers
- A flat, firm mattress that fits into the crib snugly. Make sure you can't fit two fingers between the crib and mattress.
- Two to four fitted sheets
- Four light blankets that fit into the crib
- Glider or rocking chair
- Baby monitor
- The portable changing pad that fits into a diaper bag
- Changing table with changing pad
- Plastic hangers for clothes
- Mobile
- Sunshade for car window
- Night light
- White noise machine (optional)
- Swaddle (optional)
- Diaper pail (optional)
- Toy basket (optional)

## Diapering

Changing a baby's diaper might seem like a daunting task, but you will get the hang of it. These must-haves will help you learn it faster. Here is what you need to diaper your baby.

- Diaper bag
- Two large tubes diaper cream
- Two to three large boxes unscented baby wipes
- Two to three boxes of disposable newborn diapers
- Six to ten dozen cloth diapers along with six to eight diaper covers

The last two items are per your preference. Some women don't like the thoughts of washing diapers, but some laundry companies will pick up and deliver them for you.

## Clothing

It doesn't get any cuter than teeny baby clothes. You will need to choose practical things that will keep your newborn cozy and comfortable. These are the things you need to have for your baby.

No-scratch mittens

One to three newborn hats - soft cap for winter and broad-brimmed for summer

Four to seven pairs of booties or socks. You don't need shoes until the baby begins to walk

One to three jackets or sweaters - make sure the button in the front

One to three dress-up outfits or rompers

Four to eight one-piece pajamas - try to find the ones with zippers

Four to eight nightgowns - use until the cord falls off

Four to eight pairs of pants - the footie ones are great

Four to eight shirts - kimono-style that snaps or has envelope folds at the shoulders

Four to eight onesies - snaps at the crotch and envelope folds at shoulders

Gently laundry detergent

Heavy and lightweight stroller blankets

Fleece suit or bunting bag for winter

Two wearable blankets in winter

Eight receiving blankets

Three large cotton blankets

**Bath Time**

Bath time with baby can be fun, well, after learning how to handle a slippery baby. The best way is to have the right equipment. These are what you need for your baby's bath.

- Baby lotion
- Soft washcloths
- Two to four hooded baby towels
- Baby shampoo
- Body wash
- Baby bathtub

**Health**

Never forget that babies need to be groomed, too. If your child does get sick, you will need to have the right equipment on hand. Here is what you are going to need.

- Four to six pacifiers (if you are using)
- Cradle cap brush
- Bulb syringe for suctioning mucus
- Medicine spoon or eye dropper
- Fever medication
- First aid kit
- Sterile gauze and petroleum jelly - to take care of the circumcision
- Baby thermometer
- Baby nail file
- Baby nail clippers

## Feeding

You have to be prepared to feed your newborn. This means whether you are bottle or breastfeeding, you will need a lot of things for baby's mealtime. Here are some important supplies you need to stock up on.

- Four to eight burp cloths
- Four to eight bibs
- High chair
- Nursing bra - if breastfeeding
- Breast pads - washable or disposable
- Nipple cream - if breastfeeding
- Nursing pads - if breastfeeding
- Milk storage bags - if breastfeeding
- Breast pump - if breastfeeding
- Formula - if not breastfeeding
- Dishwasher basket for baby items
- Bottlebrush
- Nipple brush
- Eight to ten nipples and bottles in both four and eight-ounce size
- Bottle sterilizer (optional)
- Bottle warmer (optional)
- Baby feeding pillow (optional)

## Baby Gear

It doesn't matter if you are relaxing at home or on the move, you are going to need to have some baby gear ready to go. At some point, you are going to need to use your arms again. Here are the things you are going to need for babies on the move.

- Playmat
- Baby bouncer
- Baby swing
- Baby carrier
- Stroller
- Convertible car seat
- Infant seat

**Dangerous Products for Baby**

While you are shopping for your baby's things, you might just think that everything on sale for babies is safe. These products were made for children, and the government has regulated them, right? Well, not always.

Some baby products have caused some injuries and death. About 40 percent of the recalls were for children's products. Before you purchase anything, check the list below to learn what products are hazardous so you can stay away from them.

- Bumbo Seats: These are dangerous because young babies can lean and fall out of them.
- Infant Bath Seats: These can fall over and cause the baby to become trapped underwater. NEVER leave baby unattended while bathing.

- Walkers: These could help your baby walk or stand before they can do it independently, but it could put your baby into dangerous positions like falling downstairs.
- Sling Carriers: These are dangerous because the baby, if not appropriately positioned, could fall out of the sling. There is also a risk of suffocations for babies under four months of age.
- Unsecured Furniture: Furniture toppling over could kill a child instantly.
- Changing Tables Without Four Sides: Your child might fall to the floor, causing serious injuries.
- Bedside Sleepers: These are also known as co-sleepers, and they let the baby sleep near mom for nursing. They could cause suffocation.
- Crib Tents: These dome or drape-style tents are used to keep a baby from getting out of their crib or play yards. The fabric could get wrapped around the baby's head and strangle them.
- Pillows: The baby could wiggle under the pillow and suffocate
- Sleep Positioners: These are used to stop the baby from getting onto their stomach or to elevate the back and head to help with acid reflux. The baby could suffocate if their face gets pushed into the positioner.

- Bumpers: Bumpers were originally designed to stop the baby from hitting their head against the crib. They could suffocate the baby.
- Drop-Side Crib: The side that moves could drop down on the baby and either strangle or suffocate the baby.

# CHAPTER 4: EXERCISE AND DIET FOR A PREGNANT WOMAN

Expectant mothers need to make sure that they have a diet that gives them the energy and nutrients they need to make sure that the baby develops and grows properly. It's also important that their body remains healthy enough for all of the changes it is about to go through.

To have a healthy pregnancy, your need to make sure that your diet is balanced and nutritious. This means that you consume the right amounts of proteins, fats, and carbohydrates, and consume many different fruits and vegetables. A diet can be impacted by health conditions, ethical beliefs, and religious requirements; it's important to check in with a doctor when planning out your pregnancy diet.

## Vegetables and Fruit

It is best if you get five servings of vegetables and fruits each day. They can be any form, including fresh, frozen, canned, dried, and juice. Frozen and fresh will provide you with the highest levels of nutrients and vitamins. It is better if you eat the fruit instead of drinking fruit juice as the natural sugars are at higher levels in the juice. Think about going with vegetable juices like carrot or wheatgrass, which is denser in nutrition.

If you are worried about getting your five a day, here are some things you can do to make it easier.

- For breakfast, have a sliced up banana and some berries in your cereal.
- Cook up different vegetables and combine them in a food processor to add them to tomato-based stews or sauces.
- Eat a salad with your evening or midday meal.
- When you want a snack, have a piece of fruit, some veggies dipped in hummus or a handful of dried fruit.

**Carbohydrate-Rich Foods**

Starchy foods rich in carbohydrates include bread, pasta, rice, and potatoes. These foods are high in energy, which means they are a very important part of a healthy pregnancy diet.

**Protein**

The best animal-source proteins for pregnant women are lean meats, chicken, and fish, as well as eggs. Those aren't the only sources of protein, so expectant mothers, especially those who follow a vegan diet, should make sure that they consume these protein sources as well:

- Nut butter, seeds, nuts, legumes, lentils, and beans have lots of iron and protein
- Soy products and tofu
- Quinoa - This is known as the "complete protein," and includes important amino acids

Research has found that expectant mothers who consumed seafood didn't suffer from as much anxiety than those who did not eat seafood. Expectant women who don't consume seafood at all was at a 53 percent great risk of having anxiety.

**Fats**

Fats should only make up 30% of your diet. Researchers at the University of Illinois found that a diet high in fat could genetically program the baby for diabetes. Consuming a diet that is overly high in fat can lead to other problems, so you must keep a balance, and the primary sources of fat should be omega-3s and monounsaturated. It's important to keep your fat intake low because it can also slow down the blood flow to the placenta. Some good fat sources include seeds, many nuts, avocados, canola oil, sesame oil, sunflower oil, peanut oil, and olive oil.

## Fiber

Wholegrain foods, like wholegrain pasta, wild rice, whole meal bread, pulses like lentils and beans, vegetables, and fruit, are rich in fiber. Women can develop constipation while pregnant, and eating plenty of fiber is a great way to reduce the risk. Research has discovered that consuming a diet high in fiber can lower the risk for hemorrhoids, which can commonly occur as the baby gets bigger.

## Calcium

Another vital mineral a pregnant woman needs is calcium. Dairy foods, like milk, yogurt, and cheese, are full of calcium. If you are vegan, you should think about consuming some of the following calcium-rich foods. Think about calcium-fortified juices and plant-based milk, as well as soynuts, kale, beans, mustard greens, okra, Chinese cabbage, collards, broccoli, bok choy, soybeans, and calcium-set tofu.

## Zinc

Zinc is also an important trace element that most of us don't even think about. Zinc plays an important part in normal development and growth, several biological functions, and cellular integrity. Specifically, it helps with protein synthesis and nucleic acid metabolism.

Since all of these are involved when it comes to cell division and growth, zinc helps the fetus grow and develop properly. Some of the best ways to consume zinc include shrimp, ham, turkey, chicken, tofu, lentils, eggs, cereals, pasta, rice, wheat germ, bran, onions, ginger, sunflower seeds, nuts, peanut butter, beans, dairy products, fish, meat, oysters, and crab.

**Iron**

Iron makes up most of your hemoglobin. Hemoglobin is the main protein and pigment of the red blood cells that carry oxygen. It is what moves oxygen throughout the body. There will be a 50% increase in the overall amount of blood in a woman's body during pregnancy. That means she requires more iron for all of the hemoglobin that she will need for the blood.

Most women start their pregnancies without an extra reserve of iron that is needed for what their body is getting ready to consume, especially after the third or fourth month. If you don't have enough stored iron, you could become anemic, and this places you at a greater risk for:

- Fatigue, depression, and irritability
- Newborn death
- Stillbirth
- Low-weight baby
- Preterm delivery

Expectant mothers who become anemic later in their pregnancy have a greater chance of losing more blood during the delivery process. The best foods to eat for more iron include:

- Whole grains
- Vegetables, particularly dark leafy ones - kale, collards, asparagus, dandelion leaves, spinach, and broccoli
- Seeds - almonds and Brazil nuts
- Legumes - peas, dried beans, kidney beans, soybeans, lime beans
- Shellfish, pork, and lamb - has some iron, but isn't as good as the other items
- Salmon
- Poultry
- Oysters
- Lean meat
- Certain cereals that are iron-fortified
- Egg yolk
- Dried fruits, like apricots
- Dried beans
- Tuna

The body doesn't as well absorb purely plant-based iron sources. If you can mix in some fish, poultry, or meat, it will improve how the body absorbs them.

## The Best Foods for Pregnant Women

Being pregnant means that you are likely going to be hungry a lot. The problem can be finding food that makes tummy and baby happy. After being told you should consume a nutritious diet while pregnant, you could be wondering what you can eat. The main thing is to make sure you stick with whole foods as they tend to have more good stuff that you need when pregnant. That said, it's okay to have a treat every now and then.

The following foods are super nutritious and should be consumed when you are pregnant. If you are allergic or averse to the foods in any way, speak with your doctor for alternative options.

- Dairy Products

While pregnant, you need to make sure you get plenty of calcium and protein to make sure your little can grow well. Dairy products like yogurt, cheese, and milk is a great source of both. In fact, dairy is the best source of calcium and contains zinc, magnesium, B vitamins, and phosphorus.

There are some varieties of Greek yogurt that also contain probiotic bacteria, which will help your digestive health. Some lactose-intolerant people can tolerate yogurt, so check with your doctor to find out if you can test it out.

- Legumes

The foods that fall under this category include peanuts, soybeans, chickpeas, beans, peas, and lentils. These are a great plant-based source of calcium, folate, iron, protein, and fiber, all things that a pregnant woman needs.

- Sweet Potatoes

Sweet potatoes can be cooked in many delicious ways, and they are also rich in beta carotene. Vitamin A is important for your baby; just make sure that you don't consume too much. Too much vitamin A from animal sources, like organ meats, can cause toxic levels of the vitamin.

Thankfully, sweet potatoes are a healthy plant-based source for fiber, and vitamin A. Fiber will help you to keep you full longer, lowers blood sugar spikes, and improves your digestion.

- Salmon

No matter how you like it, salmon is a welcomed food for a pregnant woman. Salmon is full of omega-3 fatty acids. It can help build the eyes and brain of the baby and can increase the gestational length. While you have likely heard you should avoid seafood while pregnant because of mercury levels and other contaminants, there are some fish that you can have. The main fish that have high levels of mercury include tilefish from Mexico, bigeye tuna, marlin, king mackerel, shark, and swordfish.

Salmon is also one of the very few natural sources of vitamin D, which the majority of people are lacking.

- Eggs

Eggs are the ultimate health foods as they contain every nutrient that you and your baby need. A large egg is about 80 calories, protein, fat, and several minerals and vitamins. Eggs also have choline, which is a nutrient that pregnant women need. It helps the baby's brain develop and prevents any development abnormalities of the spine and brain.

One whole egg has about 147 mg of choline, which puts you closer to the recommended amount of 450 mg per day while pregnant.

- Broccoli and Leafy, Dark Greens

There's no surprise here. We already know dark green vegetables are healthy for us. For a pregnant woman, though, they are full of nutrients that she needs. Even if you aren't a fan of them, you can hide them in some delicious dishes. They contain potassium, folate, iron, calcium, vitamin A, vitamin K, vitamin C, and fiber.

- Lean Proteins and Meat

Chicken, pork, and lean beef are great sources of protein. Pork and beef are rich in B vitamins, choline, and iron.

- Berries

In their tiny little package, berries hold a lot of healthy goodness. They contain antioxidants, fiber, vitamin C, healthy carbs, and water. Berries are also low on the glycemic scale so that they won't cause blood sugar spikes.

- Whole Grains

Unlike refined grains, whole grains are full of plant compounds, fiber, and vitamins. Think barley, wheat berries, brown rice, quinoa, and oats. Try to limit white rice, pasta, and white bread. Some, like quinoa and oats, contain a decent amount of protein.

- Avocados

Avocados are an odd little fruit in that they contain a lot of monounsaturated fatty acids. This is what makes them so rich and buttery. They also have vitamin C, vitamin E, copper, potassium, vitamin K, B vitamins, and fiber. Its healthy fats help to build tissues, brain, and skin for your baby.

- Dried Fruit

Dried fruits tend to be high in calories, various minerals and vitamins, and fiber. A piece of dried fruit has the same nutrients as fresh fruit, just without all of the water. A single serving of dried fruit can give most of your recommended daily intake of potassium, iron, and folate.

Prunes have a lot of vitamin K, fiber, and potassium. They can also help beat constipation that can come with pregnancy. Dates also have iron, potassium, and fiber.

- Fish Liver Oil

Fish liver oil comes from the oily liver of fish, most of the time, cod. It is full of DHA and EPA. These omega-3 fatty acids are essential for fetal eye and brain development.

- Water

Repeat after me, we all have to stay hydrated. This is even more important for pregnant women. With the increased blood volume, your body is going to channel the hydration to your baby. This could mean that you could become dehydrated if you don't get enough water.

**Foods Pregnant Women Should Stay Away From**

There are some foods that pregnant women should make sure that they stay away from when they are pregnant.

- Fishes High in Mercury

Fish that contain high amounts, like marlin, swordfish, and shark, need to be avoided or kept at an extreme minimum.

- Partially or Uncooked Meat

You should make sure that all meats you eat are cooked to the appropriate temperature. You should not any forms of uncooked meat and includes uncooked shellfish, as you are placing yourself at a higher risk of getting sick by a viral or bacterial contaminant, which can end up causing food poisoning. Some certain viruses and bacteria can move through the placenta and affect your baby.

- Raw Eggs

You should avoid raw or partially cooked eggs of any kind, including the whites and the yolks. Eggs need to be cooked well to prevent salmonella.

- Undercooked or Uncooked Ready-Made Meals

Ready-made meals must be cooked until they are hot all the way through. There is a risk of listeriosis, along with other infections caused by different pathogens.

- Pate

You should avoid any type of pate, whether meat or vegetable-bases. There is a high risk of a listeria infection.

- Soft Mold-Ripened Cheese

This includes Camembert, brie, or any other blue-veined cheese. Again, you have the possibility of listeria. Listeria is part of the bacteria group that is responsible for the more fatal infections for expectant mothers and their babies.

- Empty Calorie Foods

You should keep foods like candy, chips, cookies, biscuits, and cakes at a minimum. While they don't pose an infection risk, it can cause unneeded weight gain. They often have a lot of fat and sugar, and don't offer any real nutrients, and can undermine your efforts to remain healthy.

## What About Alcohol?

For decades now, the health officials have lowered the safe amount of alcohol an expectant mother can drink each week. The liver of the fetus can't process alcohol anywhere, like an adult's can. If the baby is exposed to too much alcohol, it will affect how they develop. Most doctors will tell you not to drink alcohol at all.

Some guidelines will tell you that tiny amounts each week is okay if the mother wants to consume alcohol. Heavy drinking will most definitely hurt the mother and baby. The baby can end up developing FAS, fetal alcohol syndrome, so most expectant women will choose to get rid of that risk by giving up alcohol for the duration of their pregnancy.

## What About Caffeine?

There is a chance that if an expectant mother consumes too much caffeine that the baby will have a low birth weight, which can end up causing problems for them later on in life. It also raises your risk of miscarriage. There are a lot of drinks and foods that contain caffeine other than coffee. Some examples are tea, chocolate, energy drinks, and sodas. Some flu and cold remedies have caffeine. Pregnant women need to speak with their pharmacist, doctor, or nurse before taking any type of OTC medication.

Most health professionals will tell you that you don't have to cut coffee out of your diet completely, but you should make sure that you keep your caffeine consumption to under 200 milligrams each day. Your regular cup of Joe in the morning to wake you up contains about 100 milligrams of caffeine. You may need to cut back on your intake, especially if you go with a cup of coffee all day or if you like sodas, but you can still get your caffeine fix.

**Supplements**

Pregnant women can take specific supplements to make sure that they are getting the right amounts that they need.

- Iron
- Folic Acid - It's recommended that pregnant women should take 400 mcg of folic acid a day until they reach the 12th week. Ideally, you would have already been on folic acid before getting pregnant.
- Vitamin D - It's a good idea to take a supplement of 10 mcg of vitamin D each day. Summer sunlight can also help you produce your own vitamin D. However, and you don't want to be in the sunlight too much when pregnant.
- Zinc

The one supplement that pregnant women should avoid is vitamin A supplements. Vitamin A can end up hurting the baby if too much is taken. The one exception will be if your doctor advises it for a particular reason. A doctor could find that the mother has a deficiency of vitamin A during pregnancy, so they would recommend taking a supplement.

**Exercise**

You may be pregnant, but you can still exercise. The main thing is to make sure you exercise so that it won't hurt you or the baby. As long as your health care provider says it is okay, exercising is generally safe during pregnancy. During your first prenatal care checkup, speak with your provider about what types of exercises are safe for you. If you do suffer from complications or health conditions, exercise might not be a good idea. As long as you have a healthy pregnancy, exercise will not increase your risk of premature birth, miscarriage, or low birth weight.

Healthy pregnant women should aim for 2 ½ hours each week of moderate aerobic exercise. That would equal about 30 minutes of exercise on most days. If you can't do 30 minutes at a time, try splitting up between ten minutes of exercise each day.

## Who Shouldn't Exercise?

Before we go over safe exercises for pregnant women, let's look when a pregnant woman should avoid exercise. Most of the time, your doctor will let you know if they think it is unsafe for you to exercise during pregnancy.

- "Your water breaks, preterm labor, or bleeding."

Preterm labor occurs when you give birth before the 37-week mark. Having your water break or bleeding can signal preterm labor. If this happens, you will likely be admitted to the hospital, and they will try to slow things down if at all possible

- "Having multiples along with other risk factors for preterm labor."

If you are expecting more than one, talk to your doctor to determine what kind of exercise you can do. They may ask that you don't do anything too intense or high-impact, such as running. You could still be able to do things like walking, swimming, or yoga.

- "You suffer from cervical insufficiency or a cerclage."

The cervix is the door to the uterus and is found at the very top of the vagina. An incompetent cervix, or cervical insufficiency, means that the cervix starts dilating too soon, usually with pain. This can lead to premature labor or miscarriage. If you suffer from this, or short cervix, the doctor might recommend you have a cerclage. They do this by adding a stitch to the cervix to help it stay closed.

- "You suffer from preeclampsia or gestational hypertension."

This is a high blood pressure that only pregnant women get after the 20-week mark and will go away after you have the baby.

- "You have placenta previa after 26 weeks."

This can happen if the placenta is located too low in the uterus and is blocking and area, or all, of the cervix. This can result in bleeding and other problems later on.

- "You suffer from severe anemia or certain lung or heart conditions."

If you aren't producing enough red blood cells, you could develop anemia, which means you are more likely to pass out with excessive physical activity. If you have a lung or heart condition, talk to your doctor about safe exercises.

### Safe Exercises During Pregnancy

As long as you were healthy before getting pregnant, and are used to exercising, then it is generally safe to continue your activities while pregnant. If you are a tennis player or runner or perform any other intense exercise, you could be able to continue those workouts while pregnant. As the baby grows, you might have to change the activities to make up for your growing belly.

Once you get the green light from your doctor, pick out exercises that you enjoy. If you weren't exercising before pregnancy, you could still start, and it's a good idea that you do. If you are new to fitness, go at things slowly until you are used to working out. For example, you can work out for five minutes each day until you are used to that, and then take the time up to ten, 15, and then 30 minutes.

Some safe workouts during pregnancy include:

- Strength Training

By strength training, it can help to build your muscles, which will end up making your bones stronger.

- Low-Impact Aerobics

This kind of workout doesn't put a lot of strain on the baby, which is often a better option than high-impact when you are expecting. Low-impact workouts mean that you are always going to have at least one foot on the equipment or ground. Examples are elliptical machine, stationary bike, and walking. High-impact workouts mean that you are going to end up having both feet up off of the ground at some point, which would include jumping rope, jumping jacks, and running. If you take a class, tell your teacher that you're pregnant, and they may be able to modify the workout if needed.

- Pilates and Yoga

There are prenatal yoga and Pilates classes that you can take. If you don't want to go to the gym, you can often find videos on YouTube for prenatal classes. Also, you could go to your regular class and tell your instructor that you are pregnant, and they can give you modifications.

- Swimming and Water Workouts

Water supports are very safe on the body and helps to support the baby's weight, relieving a lot of pressure off of your back. Then the movements you make will be against the resistance of the water and will help to raise the heart rate. Water workouts are great on your muscles and joints. If you have been having a lot of back pain, swimming is a great exercise to try.

- Walking

Taking a brisk 30 minute walk a day is a great workout, and it won't place any strain on the muscles and joints. This is a safe workout for anybody new to exercise.

**Exercises You Should Avoid**

Again, you should speak with your doctor about exercises you should or should not do, but in general, the following are exercises you should avoid.

- Activities that require jerky or bouncing movements that could cause you to fall. This would include skating, gymnastics, off-road cycling, downhill skiing, and horseback riding.
- Any sport that could cause you to take a hit to the belly, such as basketball, soccer, boxing, or hockey.
- Any exercise that will require you to lay flat on your back, like sit-ups. This only becomes an issue after the third month. When you lie flat on your back, the uterus places pressure on the central vein that moves blood up to the heart. When laying like this, it will cause a drop in your blood pressure, and it is going to affect the flow of blood traveling to the baby.

- Any activities that can cause you to get hit hard by the water, such as surfing, diving, or skiing.
- You should also avoid scuba diving or skydiving. Scuba diving can end up, resulting in decompression sickness. This is when dangerous gas bubbles are created within you and the baby.
- You are exercising at altitudes higher than 6000 feet unless you already live at this altitude. If you are not used to living at a high altitude, and you choose to exercise there, it can lower how much oxygen gets to the baby.
- Any exercise that can cause your body temperature to rise too high, such as exercising outside when it is hot or hot yoga. Hot yoga takes place in a room that has a temperature set to 95 to 100 degrees. This can result in hyperthermia, which can create problems for expectant women. Some studies have found that spending a lot of time in a hot tub or sauna can cause your temperature to rise too high and increase congenital disabilities.

While you are exercising, make sure that you are drinking lots of water and noticing how you are feeling. If you start experiencing any of the following while exercising, stop immediately, and contact your doctor:

- Headache
- Feeling faint or dizzy
- Chest pain, trouble breathing, or a fast heartbeat.
- Vaginal bleeding or leaking any type of fluid from the vagina.
- Muscle weakness, pain or swelling in the legs, or trouble walking. Swelling or pain in your legs could be a sign of a blood clot.
- Painful, regular contractions.
- If you stop feeling your baby moving, and you are past 20 weeks of pregnancy.

**Can Pregnancy Make Exercise Different?**

Yes, pregnancy will make things different. Your body is changing, as well as your hormones. You may notice a difference in your

- Balance - A lot of pregnant women report losing their balance more quickly.
- Body temperature - You could find that you start sweating sooner than you use to.
- Breathing - You will require more oxygen as your baby grows. As your belly grows, it will add pressure to the diaphragm, which is the main muscle that helps with your breath. While exercising, you could end up becoming short of breath.
- Energy - A lot is going on in your body right now to make sure that your baby is growing,

so you will naturally not have as much energy as you use to. You may find that you don't have the energy to do the exercises you were used to.

- Heart Rate – Your heart is working a lot harder right now, and this can affect your exercises.
- Joints – The extra hormones you have right now can cause the tissues that are supporting all of your joints to become more relaxed. Stay away from anything that could cause you to hurt or strain your joints since they don't have the support they usually do.

# CHAPTER 5: FIRST TRIMESTER: A NEW LIFE BEGINS

You may not have the obvious baby bump yet, but there is a good chance you feel pregnant. During this time, you are experiencing many hormonal changes that are prepping the body to play baby hostess. There will be quite several aches and pains, along with flatulence and fatigue. While you might not be too excited about some of these symptoms, remember that these are temporary discomforts that are helping your growing child.

The first trimester is a week on through 12. Don't know when, exactly, you got pregnant? The first thing you need to do is figure out where you are right now to figure out when you are due. It's important to remember that this due date may end up changing, mostly if your periods were irregular before you got pregnant, so just go with it.

## The Growth of the Baby

During your first trimester, the baby will start as a single fertilized cell called a zygote. Then it will become an embryo that gets implanted in the uterine wall before it turns into a bundle of limbs and systems. Organs will start to form, and the baby will begin moving. The following are some of the changes your baby will go through during this time.

- Baby's Bones

Around week six, the baby will start to grow feet, hands, legs, and arms. Toes and fingers will start to form around week ten.

- Hair and Nails

The skin will start to form between weeks five and eight, with the nail beds and hair follicles forming around week 11.

- Digestive System

By around week eight, the intestines will start to form, and your baby will have already worked its way through two sets of kidneys. The third and final set will make an appearance soon.

- Sense of Touch

The touch receptors on the baby's face will form, and is mainly on the nose and lips, by week eight. When week 12 rolls around, there will be receptors on the bottom of their feet, palms, and genitals.

- Eyesight

The optic nerves, those that pass information from your eyes to the brain and back, and the lenses start to develop around week four. The retina starts to grow at about week eight.

- Heart

At the week five mark, the tube that transforms into the hears will have spontaneous beats. At around nine or ten weeks, those beets will become more robust and regular, and you can start to hear it during your ultrasounds. This may end up happening a little later on in the pregnancy, depending on where the baby ends up being in the uterus.

- Brain

The brain will begin to develop at around week eight, and it will start to wiggle their develop arms and legs.

- Sense of Taste

At around week eight, the baby will start to form taste buds, but they will need taste pores before they can taste the surrounding amniotic fluid, which tastes like the last thing you ate.

Some other major milestones during this time include muscle formation, the development of vocal cords, and the white blood cell production that will help to fight off germs.

**Week By Week Changes**

Up until week four, your baby is about the size of a poppy seed. While it may be a tiny dot, it has many things going on with its blood vessels, one of which will become the umbilical cord. By week four, there is a better chance that you know that you're pregnant. This is also when you will need to make the big changes in giving up alcohol and smoking and going to the doctor and talking things through.

By week five, your baby is the size of a fingernail. The hands and feet are just buds, and the skull bones have started to form around the primitive brain–the outside part of the amniotic sac forms into the placenta.

By week six, your baby looks more like a tadpole than a child because the back is curved, and they have a tail. The heart started to beat on day 24. The baby has a bulge where the heart will develop. They will also have a bump where the brain is going to be. The tiny dimples on either side of the bump will become ears. You also be able to see a thick space where the eyes will form.

By week seven, your baby has started to take on alien-like qualities as their head is growing faster than their body. This is so that the brain has room to grow.

Cartilage begins to form its legs and arms. The arms will flatten out at the ends, which is where the hands will from.

By week eight, they have started to look more like a person. The baby's head will start to unfurl a little. Their arms are longer than their legs because the upper body grows faster than the rest of the body. The placenta is gearing up to care for the baby by forming "chorionic villi," which helps it to attach to the wall. This is when the baby is referred to a fetus rather than an embryo.

By week nine, your baby is now the size of a strawberry. The color of your baby's eyes have started form, and they now have eyelids. The first formation in their genitals is beginning to develop. The baby is also starting to move around, but it will still be a few weeks before you can feel the movement.

By week ten, your baby is three centimeters long, and your uterus is now about the size of a large orange. They have an upper lip now and two tiny nostrils. Their eyes can react to light. The jawbone has started to develop, and they contain their milk teeth. An ultrasound would should your baby-making little jerky movements.

By week 11, you may actually have a bit of a baby bump. You are nearing the end of your first trimester. The baby's hands now have teeny, delicate fingernails. Their toes and fingers have started to separate. Their eyes have completely closed, and they will stay that way until week 26. Their kidneys are starting to produce urine, and the stomach now as gastric juice.

By week 12, your baby is about the size of a plum. While it is still tiny, it is fully formed. From this point on, it is all about growing. The placenta has wholly developed. The cartilage skeleton is starting to become hard bone. You are officially a third of the way through your pregnancy.

**Changes Within You**

A lot is going to happen to you during your first trimester as well. Some of the most common things women experience at this time include:

- Morning Sickness - Unfortunately, somebody gave it the wrong name because it can strike at any point during the day. It will typically start around week six. Ginger ale, tea, or drops can help soothe an upset stomach. Small and frequent meals can also help. If your morning sickness is too severe, you will need to speak with your doctor to determine if there are any medications they can prescribe to help fight off the symptoms.
- Tender Breasts - Your breasts will get bigger, may tingly, and could be tender. By week six, you may start to wonder where your old boobs went.

- Mood Swings - By around week seven, you could find yourself feeling happy, sad, and happy once more. If you had depression before your pregnancy, or you feel those mood swings are something more severe, speak with your primary care provider about getting screened for depression.

As you move through this trimester, there are a lot of things that you could end up experiencing, like headaches, food aversions, metallic taste, constipation, and heartburn. Hang in there, though, once you reach the second trimester, you will find some relief. Just remember that everybody will go through things differently, so your sister or mom may have said that they peed a lot or had some cramping doesn't guarantee you will experience too.

- Weight Gain

The baby is still on the small side, which means that your weight gain is only going to be around three to four pounds during these three months. If you don't feel like eating all that much right now, you may even lose a bit of weight, and that's fine too. What's important is that your weight gain is going to pick up some much-needed steam in the last six months of your pregnancy. For now, you need to try eating several light meals during the day that are packed with nutrients, like crackers, whole grain bread, bananas, yogurt, and avocados, when you can handle it.

On the other hand, you might be feeling extra hungry. You may want to keep track of your caloric intake while you're pregnant. There is no need to eat more calories than you normally would during this time. If you do gain more weight than you need to, don't worry about it too much. Just focus on getting back to where you are supposed to be during the rest of the pregnancy.

**Symptoms to Get Checked Out**

With everything that is going on right now, there may come a time when you wonder if what you are feeling is normal or not. Most of the time, odd twinges aren't a cause for alarm. However, it's important to know the risk of a miscarriage is at the highest during this time. The following are symptoms that should warrant a call to your doctor:

- Vision disturbances
- Severe puffiness in the face and hands
- Fever over 101.5, backache, and chills
- Painful urination
- Sudden thirst
- Severe abdominal pain
- Heavy vaginal bleeding

If you experience any of those symptoms, reach out to your doctor immediately. If you can't reach your doctor quickly, head to the closest ER.

## Picking Out a Practitioner

Now that you know that you're pregnant, the next big thing is to figure out who will be a part of your pregnancy team. Those you choose will play essential roles during the pregnancy and how your delivery is going to look. With all of the choices, how can you make sure that you pick out the right practitioner to be with you throughout the pregnancy? The first thing you need to do is figure out what your priorities are. When you have a good idea of what you would like to get from pregnancy and birth, then you will have a better idea of how to pick out the right practitioner. Some things you should consider include:

- Do you want a medicated or natural childbirth?
- Where do you want to have your baby?
- Are you at a higher risk for complications?

Once you can answer these questions, then you can start looking at the different doctors who can provide you with the best service.

- OB-GYN

Over 90% of all women pick an OB-GYN. They are trained practitioners who specialize in women's reproductive health. OB-GYNs are experienced in every single part of pregnancy, which includes complications like placenta previa, multiple pregnancies, and gestational diabetes, as well as delivery, labor, and the postpartum period. They are also experienced in handling the needs of non-pregnant females, like pap smears, breast exams, and contraception. Since an OB-GYN can act as a primary care physician, it can be beneficial even after giving birth. If you wind up learning that you must have a C-section, OB-GYNs can perform one.

Going with an OB-GYN would be best if you know that you have a high-risk pregnancy, you are going to want to have an epidural, or if you already have a fantastic relationship with your current one. Remember that an OB-GYN is more likely to turn to technological or surgical interventions during the labor process.

If you are thinking about using an OB-GYN, but you don't know if you want to spend your pregnancy with your current one, now is the best time to start looking for a new one.

- Family Physician

This is a one-stop-shop that can take care of all of your medical concerns. They are training in primary, pediatric, and maternal care. This means that they can serve as an internist, OB-GYN, and, once the baby gets here, a pediatrician.

You may want to go with a family physician if you want a doctor who is always invested in every aspect of your family and health.

Remember that if complications would arid, your family physician may give you a referral to an OB-GYN.

- Certified Nurse-Midwife

CNMs are medical professionals. They have finished graduate-level school in the subject of midwifery, and the "American College of Nurse-Midwives" have certified and licensed them. They are allowed to practice in every state. CNMs have wholly and thoroughly been trained to take care of expectant women who are having a low-risk pregnancy. They want to help lower the risk of injury, trauma, and the need for C-sections by providing them with individualized care to help minimize the need for technological intervention.

They also like to use natural procedures for delivery and labor like hydrotherapy and breathing techniques. They are going to be more likely than doctors to provide breastfeeding and nutritional support. They are also able to provide regular gynecological care, and some will also help after the baby is born. While some may work within hospitals, most will work in birthing centers. You can also find a few that will perform home births. While they are less likely to use medication during birth, they can off epidurals or prescribe labor-inducing medications.

Going with a CNM could be the best choice if you want to find somebody who can help with emotional and physical needs during pregnancy. One of your priorities is to have a natural childbirth, or you are really opposed to having a C-section. CMNs have a much lower C-section delivery rate than other physicians. Or you are on a budget since CNMs tend to cost much less than an OB-GYN.

You also need to remember that you might have to go to a doctor if complications arise or if you are high-risk. There are a lot of CNMs that have a physician backup if something were to occur because they cannot perform a C-section.

- Direct-Entry Midwife

This midwife did not go through nursing training before being trained in midwifery. A DEM is an independent practitioner who was educated through midwifery school, university programs, apprenticeship, or self-study. They are more likely to do home births than the CNM, but some will work in birthing centers.

This could be the best option for you if you are 100% sure you want to have a natural home birth, and you aren't at high-risk.

It is important to remember that some of these midwives have been certified and evaluated through "North American Registry of Midwives." Still, there are some who are not certified and aren't allowed to practice legally in individual states. When you find one that is permitted to practice, certain private health insurance and Medicaid will cover their cost.

- Doula

No matter which practitioner you plan on going with, you may want to think about getting a doula. A doula doesn't have any medical training, so they will be working with a midwife or OB-GYN as a cheerleader of sorts. They are there for emotional help throughout the entire process, and after the baby is born. A doula can prove to be helpful if you need or want to have an OB-GYN, but you are afraid you won't get the emotional, hands-on support that you could get with a midwife.

As you start looking for your practitioners, make sure you ask plenty of questions and find out what their approaches are to birth procedures, prenatal care, testing, labor, and protocol for complications. When you have more information, the more ready you will be to make the best decision that will work well for you and the baby.

**Pre-Natal Testing**

You will likely be pressed, poked, and prodded several times through your pregnancy. Fortunately, most of the pre-natal tests and screenings are routine, beneficial, and pain-free. Pre-natal tests give you an accurate view of you and your baby's health and give you a chance to pick up on any complications early on. Some could even be life-saving. Other tests will provide you with information to let you know how your baby is developing, like if they have a genetic condition.

- Urine Test

This is used for the pregnancy test, but it is also used by midwives and doctors to check for two potentially dangerous complications, gestational diabetes, and preeclampsia. They are both treatable, but they can end up being dangerous if they aren't identified. Make sure you are well hydrated before all of your appointments.

- Blood Tests

At your first prenatal visit, they will do a blood test for any conditions that could affect the delivery or pregnancy. They will check for anemia, antibody titers, Rh factor, immunity to certain diseases, and hCG levels. You might also get tested for things like thalassemia, sickle cell anemia, Tay-Sachs, cystic fibrosis, and other genetic problems if you haven't been screened before.

- Pap Smear

You might have a pap smear to test for any abnormal cervical cells. You will also get screened for STIs include Chlamydia, HIV, hepatitis B, syphilis, and gonorrhea. You will be placed on antibiotics. Any other medication you need to treat infection because giving birth with an untreated disease puts your baby at a higher risk for dangerous conditions.

- Quad Screen, NT (nuchal translucency screening), NIPT (noninvasive prenatal test

This is done between 10 and 15 weeks. They screen for chromosomal abnormalities, but it does not diagnose them. NT is a specialized ultrasound, which is sometimes combined with the quad screen and NIPT, which both use a blood sample. They are not required or recommended for everybody.

- Amniocentesis and CVS

If you have a quad screen, NT, or NIPT test that shows your baby is at a higher risk for particular congenital conditions, your doctor may recommend a more invasive diagnostic test like amniocentesis or a chorionic villus sampling. These will take samples from the amniotic or placental material to check the actual genetic makeup of the baby, so this is more accurate in detecting chromosomal abnormalities, such as Down syndrome or neural tube defects.

- Glucose Screening

The glucose screening is recommended for every mom between weeks 24 and 28 to test for gestational diabetes, affecting up to 10% of all women. You will have to drink a special sugary beverage, and then you will have your blood tested. If this shows high levels of blood sugar, 140 or more, you will have to go through another test. This will require you to fast for eight hours, a blood draw, drinking another sugared drink, and undergoing at least two more blood tests over the next three hours to either confirm or rebut the diagnosis.

- Group B Strep Test

Around 25% of women have group B strep in the rectum and vagina. If you do, it is relatively harmless, but it can create an infection in the baby when they are exposed to the bacteria during childbirth. You will undergo this risk-free test toward the end of the pregnancy, which will involve having your rectum and vagina swabbed during a pelvic exam.

While undergoing tests can be stressful, the information is powerful, especially regarding your baby's health and yours. The results the tests show will give your health care provider make the best decisions for you and the baby moving forward. Most problems can be fixed before it causes a major issue.

To ease your test stress, talk to your midwife and doctor openly. Ask them what screenings and tests they are planning on conducting and when. Find out which ones are routine and which are opt-in. While most will be covered by insurance, some aren't if you aren't labeled as high-risk.

Don't ever be afraid to ask questions when you go in for a checkup. Your doctor has performed these tests thousands of times, and they might forget to fill you in on important details. Speak up and ask what the test is for and if you are confused, ask them to clarify. Your relationship with your midwife or doctor needs to be a partnership, so be active in it.

**To-Do List**

The following are some things that you need to get done or start doing during your first trimester.

If you haven't been taking them already, you should start taking some prenatal vitamins. Doing this during the first three months has proven to help reduce the risk of defects in the neural tube, such as spina bifida.

You will need to pick out a practitioner. There are many different practitioners that you can pick from when you are pregnant, just like we spoke about earlier on. So make sure that you take plenty of time to think through all of those options and decide what is going to be best for your needs.

You will need to prepare for that first visit with your OB-GYM. They will go through your medical history and give you a physical examination. You will probably be bit through a wide variety of tests, including blood work, pap smear, and urinalysis, to figure out your Rh status and blood type, as well as hCG levels and possible infections. You will also have your first ultrasound to confirm the heartbeat, make sure you are progressing well, and figure out your date of pregnancy. You may also get screened for diabetes or genetic illnesses, depending on what your family history looks like. While you will be asked a lot of questions, make sure you have some of your own. This is when you will need to find out if you can continue taking certain medications. If you haven't done so already, get help for smoking or any other question you might have.

You may also want to think about getting a genetic test. You will probably have a nuchal translucency screening, between ten and 13 weeks, to check for any congenital heart defects and Down syndrome. Based on what risks you have, your practitioner might recommend NIPT around week nine. This is a noninvasive blood screening that will check from chromosomal abnormalities. You could also get an invasive but more definitive test, such as an amniocentesis or chorionic villus sampling.

You should also take a look at your health insurance options. The price of being pregnant and having a baby will vary depending on many different factors.

You will find that it costs way more when you have no insurance to help you. That's why you need to take the time to look through your policy. Focus on things like coinsurance and premiums to help keep your overall costs as low as you can.

Coming up with a budget is also a good idea. Growing your family is the best time to reevaluate what your monthly expenses are. Learn how much it costs to have a baby, then come up with a monthly budget.

Also, make sure you take some time for you and your partner. If you feel up to it, have some sex. It's fun, a great way to relax, and it is safe.

You can also start to think about some names for your baby if you don't already have any in mind; now, it a good time to start tossing around some ideas.

Lastly, you'll want to figure out how you are going to announce your pregnancy. Think about when and how you would like to tell your family friends the good news, and if you plan on announcing it on social media. Most women will wait until after they reach their second trimester when the risk for a miscarriage is lower. You should also think about when you should tell your boss that you're pregnant. Study your company's maternity leave policy before you say anything so that you are prepared.

# CHAPTER 6: SECOND TRIMESTER: HOW YOUR BABY IS DEVELOPING

Welcome to the second trimester. This one is usually the most comfortable of all. You are going to experience some great changes. Most of the early pregnancy symptoms are going to lessen or disappear altogether. You won't feel as queasy. This means food might actually taste and smell good for the first time. You should be getting more energy, and your breast will grow, but they won't be as tender. The most amazing thing is at the end of this trimester, the bulge in your belly won't look so much like the remains of a huge lunch and more like a pregnant belly. Your second trimester begins in the 13$^{th}$ week of pregnancy and goes to the end of the 28$^{th}$ week.

## Baby's Growth

Your baby is going to be extremely busy during this trimester. By your 18$^{th}$ week of pregnancy, your baby is going to weigh about the same as a chicken breast.

They will even be able to hiccup and yawn. By about the 21st week, you should start to feel his legs and arms kick and jab you. By the 23rd week, your baby will take its cue from you and begins to put on weight. They will probably double their weight during the next four weeks. Once you reach the end of these three months, your baby will be about two pounds.

Some other things are happening this trimester, too:

- Brain: Other than being in control of your baby's kicks and heartbeat, by 26 weeks, their brain will begin blinking their eyelids.
- Heart: By week 17, the baby's heart isn't just beating spontaneously because their brain is in control of their heartbeat. By the 20th week, the heartbeat should be able to be heard through a stethoscope. By the 25th week, capillaries start forming so they can carry blood throughout the body.
- Senses: The baby's eyes and ears are moving into the right position. By the 22nd week, their senses are developing. This means they are beginning to hear, see, and smell. Their eye is starting to open.
- Digestive System: The baby's digestive system was entirely formed by the end of the first trimester. The baby is beginning to swallow and suck, preparing themselves for living outside of the womb. They can even taste the food that you eat through the amniotic fluid. This can influence their food

preferences once they are born. This is another reason you need to eat healthy foods during your pregnancy. Baby's waste systems are working hard even though they are still getting all their nutrients through your placenta, all of that swallowing means they will be peeing, too.

- Nails, Skin, and Hair: By the 16th week, the baby's first tiny hairs begin to grow. By the 22nd week, their eyebrows and eyelashes have grown in, too. Their skin is covered in lanugo, a "fur coat" that keeps them warm until they build more fat during the third trimester. By the 19th week, vernix caseosa or a greasy layer of dead skin cells and oils that protect their skin from the amniotic fluid that is acidic. The baby will shed all of this before birth.

### Week By Week Changes

By week 13, your baby is growing extremely fast. You might hear their heartbeat at one of your checkups. They weigh about 25 grams. Even though you won't feel them move, they are dancing around in you. Their hands will find their way into their mouth, and they might yawn. They only sleep for a few minutes at a time but will soon start sleeping longer. Their reproductive organs have formed inside their body, and a small penis might be beginning where a small bump was before.

By week 14, your baby is about the size of a kiwi fruit. They will be about 85mm from the top of its head to the bottom. The baby has begun swallowing some amniotic fluid. This travels through their system just like ours. If you have a midwife, they can use a fetal heart rate monitor to check its heartbeat. They just place it on your stomach, and you can hear the heartbeat. If you have an app that says it can monitor your baby's heartbeat, don't trust them as most are known to be misleading and dangerous. Hearing the heartbeat could be a special moment during your pregnancy, and it might make your baby feel more real.

By week 15, your baby is the size of an apple. They can hear sounds now, and they might be able to hear you; the sound of your heartbeat comforts them. They may be able to sense the bright lights outside the tummy. Your baby might begin getting hiccups now. Later on in your pregnancy, you should be able to feel their little flutters when they get the hiccups.

By week 16, your baby is the size of a lemon. Have you been feeling flutters? Maybe something like a bubbling sensation? This might be your baby moving around. Don't worry if you haven't; it is still early. Your baby's nervous system is still developing, and they can flex their tiny muscles. They can make fists, and they might even pull on their umbilical cord. If you have an ultrasound, you might see them squinting or frowning.

By week 17, your baby will be about 12 cm long and weigh about 150 grams. Your baby bump is getting larger. Your baby is about the size of an orange. Your baby's face now has eyebrows and eyelashes. They already have their unique fingerprint. Before now, your baby's head was always larger, but now, their body is beginning to fill out, and the proportions are beginning to even out. Your baby can move their eyes even though their eyes are still shut. They will not open them back up until week 26. The bones in their feet are starting to harden. The placenta is still growing so it can handle all your baby's needs.

By week 18, your baby is about the size of a bell pepper. Once your baby is born, you might have people tell you to use noise to help them sleep. The main reason this work is because they are used to this noise. The womb is not at all silent. By 18 weeks, your baby can hear sounds around them and may respond to loud noises or music.

By week 19, your baby is as long as a banana, and you should be able to feel them move. You might feel them kicking or prodding you. They are growing fast and gaining a lot of weight, but they don't have a lot of fat on their body. They are very wrinkled and won't begin filling out until the last few weeks of the pregnancy. Although your baby won't get their first tooth until they are about six months, they are forming their second teeth behind the first ones right now.

By week 20, if your baby were to stand up, they would be about 26 cm tall, about the length of a piece of A4 paper. Their skin is covered in a creamy, white substance called vernix. This will protect their skin. If you see your baby during an ultrasound, they might be sucking their thumb. They are practicing their sucking, and this is important for when they begin nursing.

You have reached week 21, and you are halfway there. Your baby's hair is growing, and they are beginning to look more like a baby that you will meet a bit later. Your baby is about the length of a carrot and weighs about 350 grams. Even though the ears were formed earlier, they will be able to hear now. They will be able to recognize sounds like the people around you and your voice. This is the time to sing or talk to your baby if you want to. You can encourage others to do so, too. It's an excellent way to get everyone involved. Their hair is getting thicker and showing signs of what color it will be.

By week 22, your baby weighs about one pound. They will weigh more than the placenta from here on out. They are about the size of a bag of sugar. Their taste buds are developing, and they have been busy practicing swallowing, getting ready for their new life. Everything you eat can affect the flavors your baby likes after they are born. This is why you need to eat healthy foods. Your baby's lungs are developing rapidly. However, they can't breathe while in the womb; they practice their breathing movements for their new life. They are getting all the oxygen from your blood, and that's all they need.

By week 23, your baby is the size of a large mango. They will probably get hiccups more often, and you might feel their tiny jerks when it happens. They will also begin sucking their thumb. If you feel bubbles and fluttering from your baby, you have probably felt some jabs and kicking too. These will get more noticeable over the next few weeks ad the baby grows bigger and gets stronger. You might notice that when you try to sleep, your baby gets active, but when you are moving about, the baby goes to sleep. This is the best time to get to know your baby's routine. By doing this, you will begin understanding your baby's habits and will know when something is wrong.

By week 24, your baby is about the size of an ear of corn. You might have noticed they are getting into a pattern of waking and sleeping. When you are in bed, feeling all relaxed, you might realize they are wriggling and awake. Your baby is now "viable." This means there is a chance that they will survive if they were to be born now. Any baby born now would need some help from a neonatal unit because their body isn't mature enough to handle the outside world.

By week 25, your baby will respond to sound, touch, and light. You may even notice them kicking or jumping in response to loud noises. Your baby is frequently peeing, and this goes into the amniotic fluid. Their lungs, digestive system, and brain are developed but not yet matured. They will still develop as the pregnancy progresses.

By week 26, your baby is beginning to open and close their eyes now. Their eye color is probably blue. A little while after they are born, they will change to the color they will stay. Your baby will measure at about 35 cm from the top of their head to the bottom of their heels. This is about the length of your forearm. They are about the length of a zucchini. Your uterus still has a lot of room, and you can feel your baby move around a lot. Over the next few months, your baby will be putting on more muscle and fat and begin looking less skinny and wrinkly and more like a little angel.

By week 27, your baby is about the size of a head of cauliflower. You are almost at the end of the trimester, and your family might be able to feel your little one's movements, too. If your baby were to stretch out completely, they might be 37 cm long. They are a tangle of limbs that take up a lot of room in your womb. Their heart rate had slowed down to around 140 beats per minute. Even though this is very speed compared to yours, their heartbeat can be heard through a stethoscope, and your significant other might be able to hear it if they lay their ear on your belly, even though it might be hard finding the correct spot.

By week 28, your baby is about the size of an eggplant and weighs about one kg. They are taking up more space, and as the weeks move on, you might begin feeling a bit tired and uncomfortable. Your baby will have periods of activity and sleep. You will probably be aware of these and have noticed they are settling into a normal pattern. Notice these patterns because it will help you see if their movements slow down. If this were to happen, you need to call your doctor immediately.

**Your Body Changes**

During this trimester, there will be some pregnancy symptoms that are still going to be there, like constipation and heartburn. Some others might pop up as your belly grows and the hormones rise, including:

- Hemorrhoids or Varicose Veins: Hemorrhoids are one kind of varicose vein that should go away after giving birth if you didn't already have them before you got pregnant.
- Lower Abdomen Pain: This is also known as "round ligament pain" as the ligaments supporting the belly begin stretching to support the belly's bigger size.
- Dizziness: This can be caused by lower blood pressure because of all the extra blood your body has to pump. Be easy on yourself, eat lots of small meals, and drink lots of fluids to reduce the symptoms.

- Leg Cramps: These typically begin during the second trimester and go through the end of the third. These happen because of the weight and hormones, but it might be from a shortage of magnesium and calcium. Make sure you continue to eat healthy, well-balanced meals.
- Sensitive Gums: You might also have some bleeding gums. Make sure you visit the dentist if your gums turn bright red and bleed extremely easily. This might be a sign of gingivitis.
- Feet and Ankles Swelling: This is usually experienced by about three out of every four women who are pregnant. This can begin around the 22nd week and last until you deliver. To lessen some of the swelling, stay active, if possible. When you aren't moving, keep your feet elevated. Try not to sit or stand for too long and sleep on your side.
- Congestion: Even though blood flow has increased to the mucus membranes in your body, you might realize that you are snoring. Some OTC medications are safe for you to use during pregnancy.
- Leaking Nipples: You might notice some yellow stains on the inside of your bra. This is just a small amount of colostrum, which is the first milk that you will produce. Your breasts could begin producing milk at 14 weeks. You

can use absorbent breast pads to keep this from getting onto your clothes.

- Nosebleeds: you may have some nosebleeds due to the hormonal changes, and the increased blood in your body can put more pressure on your blood vessels in your nose, which could cause them to break. This is common but if it persists, call your doctor.
- Thrush: This is a type of fungal infection. If you see any symptoms, call your doctor.

These are temporary and totally normal, just like the feelings of frustration, forgetfulness, irritability, and apprehension. You are looking completely plump but not completely pregnant.

There might some changes in the bedroom, too. Being pregnant can cause problems with your sex life since both of you are going to have to handle the changes in your body, and all of the symptoms can end up killing the mood. Some women might have an increased sex drive than they had before, with all of the blood being fed into the right areas. Just make sure you and your partner do the following: Communication is vital to avoid resentment. Talk to your partner through any dry spells. Sex isn't going to hurt the baby or emotionally scar them. They might actually enjoy some rolling and rocking.

## Gaining Weight

In the upcoming months, you will begin gaining a lot of weight. Your appetite is probably going to increase or show up if you had a lot of nausea during your first trimester. This is needed to support the growing baby. If you began your pregnancy at a normal weight, you should gain about a pound each week for a total of about 14 pounds in this trimester alone.

## When to See Your Doctor

For the most part, after you reach this trimester, everything else will be smooth sailing, but there are some things that you need to keep an eye out for and contact your doctor if you experience any of them. The most important one to look for is heavy vaginal bleeding, fever over 101.5, and lots of abdominal pain.

Watch out for signs of gestational diabetes. This usually begins about the 24 or 28th week. Some signs are snoring, extreme fatigue, copious and frequent urination, extreme thirst. Call your doctor if you have sudden weight gain, lots of swelling in the hands, face, changes in your vision. These could be signs of preeclampsia.

## Second Trimester Survival Kit

As your body continues changing during this time of your pregnancy, several items can help you feel and look your best. Some might help you get more sleep, others will help you stay hydrated, and others are just fun.

This checklist has everything you are going to need to get through the second trimester easily:

- Maternity Clothes

Now that your bump is beginning to show, you are going to need to invest in a few pieces of maternity clothes. All moms need to have a fun T-shirt to announce and celebrate your pregnancy.

- Belly Butter

As the baby grows, your belly will stretch, and you might experience some discomfort and itching. Using belly butter regularly can help with this discomfort. It might prevent stretch marks from happening, too.

- Belly Band

By this trimester, you have probably outgrown a few pairs of your favorite pants, and most of your shirts might look like crop tops on you. Belly bands can help add some length to your tops and hide your unbuttoned pants so you won't feel as exposed while keeping your clothing costs down.

- Comfortable Bras

Your breasts might grow a full size or even larger during your pregnancy. This is why it is so important that you have the right support for them. Finding a comfortable bra that is properly fitted can help relieve the pressure from your ever-growing breasts. A good pick would be a nursing bra, as it will come in handy if you plan on breastfeeding.

- Epsom Salt

Most moms-to-be will experience leg cramps during the second trimester. These can steal that precious sleep that you have been missing. An excellent way to relieve this is to take a warm bath with Epsom salts before going to bed. This can prevent cramps, but a warm bath can relax you.

- Nasal Strips

Nasal congestions will begin to kick in during this trimester. This makes it more likely that you will begin snoring. That same congestion could make getting a good night's sleep hard to come by. If you do start snoring, you need to grab a pack of nasal strips.

These make it easier for you to breathe without taking decongestants that haven't been approved for pregnant women.

- Pregnancy Pillow

While your belly gets bigger, you will experience some discomfort while trying to sleep. Body pillows can give you're the support your growing baby bump needs, so you can get the sleep you need before the baby gets here. If the body pillow is too large for you, a pregnancy pillow wedge could support your stomach.

- Water Bottle

I know you are probably making a hundred plus trips to the bathroom, but you have to stay hydrated. It is vital to your baby's health and your health. A large water bottle could help you get your eight glasses each day in style. Don't worry, most of the "glass" ones are shatterproof.

- Resistance Bands

A healthy, strong mom equals a healthy baby. Plus, being fit might mean less time spent in labor, and it can also help speed up your postpartum recovery. Now that your morning sickness is beginning to go away, it is the perfect time to start some gentle strength-training exercises to help you through delivery. If your doctor says its okay, using resistance bands is very effective.

# CHAPTER 7: THIRD TRIMESTER: BABY IS GETTING READY FOR BIRTH

You have finally made it into the home stretch. You have entered into the last three months of pregnancy, and you are likely super excited to meet your little bundle of joy. The third trimester starts at week 29 and ends at week 40, or once you give birth. You have a good chance of going into labor a week or so early or later. Around 30% of all births will go beyond the 40-week mark. There are some tricks women have tried to induce labor, but you won't officially be considered overdue until you reach week 42. This is when your doctor may start talking about inducing labor if things don't get started on its own.

## Baby's Growth

Your little one is getting ready to get a whole lot bigger during these last three months. They go from about two and a half pounds and 16 inches long around the 28-week mark, to between six and nine pounds and upwards of 22 inches long by week 40.

With its increase in size and decrease in living space, you will likely experience some serious pokes and kicks to the gut.

- Bones - as their cartilage changes to bones during months seven and eight, the baby will be getting their calcium needs from you, so make sure you are getting plenty of calcium.
- Nails, hair, and skin - by week 32, their skin has become opaque. Fat will continue to accumulate as the baby sheds its vernix and lanugo.
- Digestive system - during the last few weeks, the baby's first poop is going to start forming and will be made up of lanuga, vernis, and blood cells.
- Five senses - they developed their touch receptors during week 29 or 30. Then, by week 31, they will have all of their five senses. They will be able to listen to your voice, taste the foods you eat and perceive light and dark.
- Brain - the brain is growing faster than ever now and is testing out its ability to regulate the baby's temperature, dreaming, and blinking.

At around the 34-week mark, the baby should turn southward and settle with into a heads-down, bottom-up position. If your baby chooses to be stubborn and remain in the breech position, the doctor will likely to manually move them at around week 37.

**Week By Week Changes**

By week 29, the baby is about the size of butternut squash. There are some surprising symptoms that you can experience during pregnancy, and the main one during this time is leaky breasts. Colostrum, a thin, yellowish fluid, can be expelled, but this is simply a precursor to breast milk. Most of the time, it will only be a couple of drops, if any, but if it becomes heavier, using nursing pads in your bra can help. This fluid houses many antibodies that can help to fight off infection and to build up resistance to a lot of common diseases for the baby's first few days out of the womb. So even if you aren't planning on breast-feeding for months, you should consider nursing them a couple of days so that the baby can use this nutritional head start.

By week 30, your baby is the size of a large head of cabbage. Stretch marks aren't the only common side effect of expanding skin. Around 20% of moms will experience itchy skin. You can talk to your doctor about this, and they may recommend ointments or antihistamines, but a lotion with oatmeal can also help. Around half of moms-to-be will get stretch marks, usually around the sixth and seventh months. No matter what some products say, you can't prevent them. They won't ever disappear completely, but they will fade. Some prescription creams and laser treatments can help to lighten them up, but this should not be done until you are several months postpartum, or at least until you are done nursing.

By week 31, your baby is the size of a coconut. All babies are different, even during this stage, so your baby will have their own movement patterns. This is a good time to become aware of the patterns. Then, if you notice a significant change or reduction in the movements, you can contact your doctor or midwife immediately.

By week 32, your baby is the size of a cantaloupe. Since the uterus has now moved to around five inches above the belly, the baby has started to press more on your organs. You can expand some urine leakage, breathlessness, and heartburn to increase during the last little bit. This can also affect your appetite. Some mothers will notice their nausea coming back.

By week 33, your baby is the size of a pineapple. The nervous system in your baby is now fully developed. Their bones are also getting firmer at this point. Don't worry about giving birth to something as big as a pineapple because their skull is designed to make it easier for the baby to leave the birth canal. It stays soft and in separate pieces until after they are born to move and protect the brain.

By week 34, your baby is the size of a large melon. Feeling like your body couldn't possibly grow anymore? Luckily, your weight gain will usually plateau or slow a bit around this time. Still, you probably aren't able to see your shoes, you might actually find it a bit more comfortable to wear a bra for the first time while you are sleeping, and your new outie bellybutton might cause some self-consciousness. You are going to be back to your old self in just a few weeks, along with an amazing baby.

By week 35, your baby is the size of a honeydew melon. All of the extra fat that your baby has started to build up helps to regulate their body temperature once they are born. If your baby is a boy, his testicles are getting ready to drop from the abdomen into the scrotum. You may also find that you are due for another bra, as your breasts are still growing.

By week 36, your baby is the size of a large cabbage and weighs around six pounds. Your baby's living space has shrunk significantly. However, this is not going to slow down there, kicking. If at any point you feel a reduction in their movement, get in contact with a doctor or midwife. Your baby's lungs stay deflated until they are born and take their first breath of air. This is why there is no risk of drowning when you have a water birth. If the baby is born now, they would be considered moderately premature.

By week 37, your baby is the length of a stalk of Swiss chard. Sex is probably the furthest thing from your mind right now, but some experts believe it to be beneficial, and most will agree that it is completely harmless. The cervix is engorged with blood and is very sensitive at this point, so you might notice spotting after sex. If you find that the spotting persists or you see bright red discharge, contact your doctor. Your baby is also considered full-term at this point.

By week 38, your baby is the length of a stalk of rhubarb. The thoughts of your water breaking at any time now are probably plaguing your mind, and you may be thinking up a bunch of embarrassing public scenes. Rest assured, though, that it likely won't happen that way. Most women will feel the wetness running down their leg and not a sudden gush of water, so you should be able to get to the bathroom in time to save yourself from an embarrassing situation.

By week 39, your baby is the size of a small watermelon; you like to feel like the size of a whale. Fewer than five percent of women will give birth on their due dates. This means that your baby could be born in just a few hours, or it could be another two weeks. But you are so attuned to the chance of labor that each twinge you experience will have you jumping. Labor can start in many different ways. It could be mild cramps, most common, water breaking, or if you have scheduled a C-section or induction, a drive to the hospital. Labor will then happen in three stages.

By week 40, you are ready for your baby to get here, and they are about the size of a pumpkin. This is the week your baby is due, and if you are lucky, you will get to meet them soon. You will soon be experiencing your first contractions. They will be fast and furious once you reach active labor, and they can last a minute each. You are going to feel pain moving throughout your stomach, upper thighs, and lower back. This will be something you have never felt before, and everybody will deal with it in their own way.

That said, you may still be pregnant when week 40 ends, and that means you are starting week 41. Babies are born on their terms, not yours, and can come anywhere from 38 and 42 weeks. Week 40 is chosen as your due date because it is the midpoint of this period.

Some women choose to schedule their pregnancy instead of letting nature take its course. This means that you will go to the hospital whenever you are scheduled to, assuming the baby hasn't decided to make an earlier arrival. Scheduled childbirth can either be a C-section or an induction. An induction means you will still deliver vaginally, you will just be giving something to induce labor, such as prostaglandin gel to soften up the cervix, or you will get an IV drip of Pitocin to start contractions. For those who go into labor on their own, they should notify their doctor or midwife.

And if you are still pregnant at week 42, that's okay. It shouldn't be too much longer. You aren't technically overdue until after week 42. If you do reach week 43, the doctor may want to talk about inducing the labor or breaking your water.

### Your Body Changes

You are likely to feel a lot of fetal activity at this point. You will also notice that your bump is growing a lot bigger now. Some other things you may notice are:

- Abdominal aches - the round ligaments, those that support the lower abdomen, stretch to accommodate your belly, and this could cause sharp pains or cramps. The best thing to do is to take it easy.
- Fatigue - you are probably going to feel pretty zapped now because of everything your body is going through. Eat well, and often, stay as active as you can, and figure out how to get some sleep.
- Heartburn - during the last couple of weeks of pregnancy, the uterus will press on the stomach and push its contents up, causing a persistent burn. If the heartburn is getting to you, speak with your doctor about some safe antacids you could take.
- Braxton Hicks contractions - this is how your body gets ready for labor. These are practice contractions that are irregular and happen randomly.
- Varicose veins - you may notice a few of your veins bulging in the lower half of your body because of the excess blood you have coursing through you. The great this is, if they

weren't there before you got pregnant, they would likely go away once you give birth.

- Stretch marks - these are tiny tears in your skin, which appear once the skin is stretched to the limit. Moisturize to minimize them.
- Backache - relaxin, a pregnancy hormone, will loosen your joints, and your belly is going to pull your center of gravity forward, and this can create an achy back. This is why you should put your feet up as much as you can.
- Crazy dreams - due to all of those hormones, you may notice that your dreams are more vivid the closer you get to your due date. These usually aren't anything to worry about, so don't worry about them too much.
- Clumsiness - hormones are going crazy, your belly is keeping you off balance, and you forget everything. This is all normal, so just try to keep a sense of humor about it all.
- Lack of bladder control - if you laugh, you pee. The extra weight that is on the pelvic floor causes you to have problems keeping yourself dry. Add Kegels to your routine.
- Leaky breasts - things are gearing up for your baby.

**When to See Your Doctor**

As your due date starts to approach, you might experience signs of false labor. The following are some real signs of labor that you need to keep an eye out for to know when to go to the doctor.

- Lightening - this is also called dropping and is when the baby moves into the birthing position. You can notice this around week 36 when you find yourself waddling.
- Bloody show - this is a stringy mucus tinged pink or brown discharge and is a sure sign of labor. You might also notice the discharge of the mucous plug.
- Labor contractions - when compared to Braxton Hicks, these will get stronger instead of diminishing the more you move.
- Water breaking - this is the ultimate sign that you are in labor.

However, if at any point during these last three months you experience heavy vaginal bleeding, 101.5 fever or higher, sudden weight gain, severe abdominal pain, preterm labor signs, or any other worrisome signs, contact your doctor immediately. It is better to go with your instincts and stay safe when you are pregnant.

## Finding a Comfortable Sleeping Position

One of the biggest problems women have with their growing bellies is getting comfortable in bed. Your regular sleeping positions won't be all that helpful during pregnancy. As you know, your body is going through quite a few changes during pregnancy, and this disrupts sleep.

You knew that you would be facing sleepless nights once the baby was born, but you never realized that they were going to start before the baby arrived. Depending on where you are in your pregnancy, everything from scary dreams to morning sickness to restless leg can affect your shut-eye.

One thing you should do as soon as you find out that you are pregnant is to change your sleep schedule. Take naps as often as you can because you need extra rest during this time. It's also not a bad idea to keep Saltines in your nightstand to help queasiness during the night.

The best position to choose while pregnant is to sleep on your side. Sleeping on your left side is even better. This will increase the number of nutrients and blood that can reach your baby and the placenta.

You don't even have to sleep completely on one side. By using a pillow, you can make yourself think you are in your favorite position. As you are on your back, put a pillow under your right hip. This will help to tilt the uterus so that blood can freely flow, but it will keep your back and upper chest flat.

If you have back pain, the side position with a pillow under the abdomen works well. If you have heartburn, you can use extra pillows to prop your upper body up. During the last first weeks of pregnancy, when you may be having shortness of breath, you can try lying on your side or propped up a bit of some pillow.

While this might not sound that great, especially if you are usually a stomach or back sleeper, but you should try them. You will likely find that they work pretty well. Remember that you don't always stay in one position during the night, and changing positions is perfectly fine.

Full-body and wedge pillows are the best friends of a pregnant woman. You can also choose to sleep in a recliner or comfy armchair if you cannot sleep in the bed.

If you find that you are particularly restless during the night, try working out during the day to help you feel sleepier. Ensure you don't exercise during a couple of hours before bed, since it can end up ramping you up.

If your bladder keeps you up, avoid drinking liquids during the two hours before bed. If your mind doesn't stop worrying about things, talk to somebody or journal for a bit.

There are some positions that you shouldn't sleep in, though. For one, sleeping on your back can create more backaches, breathing problems, issues with the digestive system, low blood pressure, hemorrhoids, and decrease the circulation to the baby and heart. When you are on your back, it causes the abdomen to rest on your major blood vessels and intestines. Sleeping on your stomach becomes pretty much impossible the farther along you are in your pregnancy.

Overall, it is a good idea to make a full routine to get your body ready for bed. Start by taking a warm bath and get a relaxing leg massage. Avoid that last cup of water and have your pillows ready. Don't bring things into the bedroom like bills, so that all you focus on is sleep or sex. A little meditation and some aromatherapy can help out as well.

### Playing Music to Your Baby in the Womb

Babies can learn from within the womb. This learning simply means that the baby is able to create a familiarity with something. In a 2013 study, they found that babies who played the same song while in the womb would calm down when the song was played once they were born.

But this doesn't mean that you have to run out and buy learning CDs and belly beds to help your kid learn multiple languages. Most brain development will happen outside of the womb. That means you should save the language lessons until later.

Your baby will develop ears during week three of gestation, but they don't work until week 16. While we all understand that the fetus can actively listen around week 24, ultrasounds have found that the fetus can hear and respond to sounds by week 16.

But you can still play your baby some Mozart or Beethoven. Anything that you find relaxing and you enjoy doing while pregnant will positively affect your baby. If you sing along with the music, your baby will hear and feel your voice and create a stronger bond with how you sound and melodies that you like.

The good news is, there isn't one type of music that is better than the other. Doctors do say that simple tunes work best, but pretty much anything you like will be fine. The key is to make sure you listen to things because you like them.

Now, the womb is a boisterous place to be. The stomach makes noises, your heart is beating, and your lungs are filling with air. On top of all of that, your voice is also amplified through the vibration of your bones as the sound of your voice travels throughout your body.

That said, while you are pregnant, you need to keep the outside volume of things to around 50 to 60 decibels. This is equal to the volume of a normal conversation. This means you shouldn't put headphones over your belly. According to doctors, by the time the sound coming out of the earphones reaches the baby, it will be very loud, which you want to avoid.

You are free to go to a concert every once in a while or go to the movies now and then, but regular exposure to extreme volumes is something that most doctors will warn against. Loud concerts should be avoided entirely after 18 weeks.

With those warnings aside, you should sign, dance, and enjoy music throughout your pregnancy, and your baby is going to love it too. One of the main benefits of listening to music while pregnant is because of stress levels. High stress in moms will harm fetal development. Singing and music soothes the expectant mother and baby and will contribute to a happy and healthy baby later on. Music will also start the all-important prenatal bond. When you relax to music or sing lullabies, it will send out calming chemicals through your body and through the placenta, which will help with relaxation and bonding.

Listening to various types of music will also encourage early brain development because music will facilitate neuron connections. Experiencing and listening to music helps to stimulate the baby's brain and will assist with the growth of different brain structures.

**To-Dos**

During these last three months, you should make sure that you keep track of the fetal movement. From around 28 weeks and on, you will want to keep up with how often the baby kicks you and notice any changes inactivity, especially during the last month.

Keep an eye on your weight as well. Pregnancy weight gain should pick up some speed during this time and then taper off as you get closer to your due date. If you aren't gaining enough, or you have gained more than you should, speak with your doctor to adjust your diet.

Continue to move, as long as your doctor tells you it's okay. Make sure you stay safe and that you are still doing pregnancy-safe exercises.

Schedule all of the checkups your need. Expect to have glucose levels test, anemia, and group B strep during the seventh and eighth months. During month nine, you will undergo an internal examination of the cervix to see if effacement and dilation have started. If you have been told you are "high-risk," the doctor could schedule a nonstress test or biophysical profile during the last couple of weeks of pregnancy to ensure things are going to correctly

Take a tour of the hospital or birthing center. If you've not already done this, month seven is the best time to visit the place where you plan on giving birth.

Pick out your baby's pediatrician. Speak a few different candidates and ask them the same questions at around week 32, and then choose the one you like the most.

Get that baby gear ready. Ensure you have the essentials that you are going to need for the baby, especially a stroller, crib, changing table, baby monitor, and car seat, which you are going to have to have to get the baby home from the hospital. You should also think about taking the car seat to either be installed or inspected by a professional

Get educated about birth. Besides going to your regular childbirth class, which teaches you what to do during the birthing process, you may want to think about taking an infant CPR class.

Get ready for breastfeeding. Read about the ways to breastfeed and why you should before the baby gets here, and if you can, think about taking a breastfeeding class. Don't hesitate to reach out to a lactation consultant or doula for help.

Learn how the various stages of labor progress. Make sure that you are ready for the birth of the baby and know what will go on during early, active, and transitional labor, as well as what it will be like to deliver the baby and placenta.

Think about how you want to manage labor pains. Are you going to want an epidural or some other medication for the pain? Are you thinking about having a natural birth, possibly a water birth? This is the time to start talking about your options with your practitioner.

Check on your birth plan. This is all of the details about what you want for your birth, such as epidural, who cuts the umbilical cord, and all of the other important details. Just keep in mind, your birthing plan does not go as you plan. You have to be flexible.

Get the nursery ready. Get the things you will need for the nursery, and don't forget to stock up on the bottle, pacifiers, wipes, diapers, baby clothes, and formula if you plan not breastfeeding.

Think about commemorating the baby bump. Get some professional pregnancy pictures taken. You can also get a cast made of your bump if you would like.

Fill up your fridge and freezer. In the week or so before you are due to give birth, whip up some meals to freeze so that you won't have to think about cooking during the baby's first few weeks of life.

Get your hospital bag packed. You should pack light, but don't forget to pack some comforts from home that you might want while at the hospital.

Get ready for your baby's first year of life. Learn more about everything your baby will go through during that time. There is a lot to look forward to.

# CHAPTER 8: LABOR

There will come a time in your pregnancy when all you can do is wait. You have read all of the books, the nursery has been decorated, and the car seat is installed correctly. You're now within the 37 to 42 weeks of pregnancy phase, and you can give birth at any moment. There is no way to know exactly when you will give birth, and this unknown can create a lot of anxiety.

For first-time moms, it can be hard to figure out when you are in labor. A lot of women will head to the hospital because of Braxton Hicks contractions. To know for sure if your contractions are the real deal, wait a bit before going to the hospital and see if they become stronger and last longer and come closer together. That tells you labor is afoot.

Even if you are in labor, it can take a bit to be sure, so during the early stages, you are better off to stay at home so that you are in a comfortable place. First-time moms should expect to be in labor anywhere from 12 to 14 hours. With each subsequent pregnancy, the delivery usually goes faster.

When it is time to get to the hospital or birthing center, keep in mind that most things don't normally go as you planned. You might be told you can't get the epidural you wanted, or you could end up having to have an emergency C-section. It is a good idea to know how you would like things to go, but you also need to make sure that you can be flexible for the unexpected.

Labor is a personal experience and will be different for every woman and every pregnancy that she has, but this is what could happen.

**First Stage: Effacement and Dilation of Cervix**

Your doctor will probably let you know when you should call them or head to the hospital. Still, you usually do this when contractions start happening at regular intervals, like every eight or ten minutes, and they continue to grow closer. Another indication would be the rupture of membranes, which is a fancy way of saying your water broke, losing the mucus plug, and passing blooding discharge, also called show.

Not every single woman is going to experience all of these signs, so if you aren't sure, then give your doctor a call.

- Early Phase: Cervix dilates to three or four centimeters

This early phase of the labor process is sometimes lovingly referred to as "the entertainment phase," because this is a good time to try to focus on other things so that you can help to pass the time without staying focused on what is to come. As long as the contractions stay "mild" and are spaced at least five minutes apart, most women will stay at home at this point and keep in close contact with their doctor or midwife.

It is best to enjoy the comfort of your familiar surroundings as staying relaxed is more critical during this time. The more comfortable you can stay, the smoother delivery will go. If you go into early labor during the day, try doing some simple routines at home. Try to keep yourself occupied while also saving your energy. Drink lots of water and eat plenty of small snacks. Make sure that you and your partner are keeping track of your contractions. If your early labor starts during the night, it is best to get as much sleep as possible. If you can't get to sleep, then get up a do some light activities, such as making lunch for the next day, packing a bag, or some light cleaning.

Typically during this phase, contractions will be a mild and bit irregular and come anywhere from five to 30 minutes apart and will last around 30 to 45 seconds. You could notice a pinkish discharge, and you might feel a bit of discomfort in the abdomen. Your water could break during this time, or it can happen later on, or it may have to be broken by your doctor.

This stage normally lasts around six to ten hours for first-time moms, but it can last two to five hours if you have had a child before. Your cervix should efface and dilate to four centimeters.

These contractions normally last between 30 and 60 seconds and will start at 20 minutes apart and work towards five. Look for contractions that will continue even if you start walking around that becomes stronger, and that begins in your back and spread around to your front.

You can also experience contractions that feel like an ache in your lower back, tightening and pressure in the pelvic area or menstrual cramps. Your water may break at this point, and it can happen at any time during the first stage of labor.

When you have a contraction, try to notice the following:

- They are getting closer together.
- They are lasting longer.
- They are keeping a regular pattern.
- They are growing more intense.

If your water does break, notice the following:

- The time your water broke.
- The odor of the fluid.
- The color of the fluid.

- Active Phase: Cervix has dilated from four to seven centimeters

This is when things get serious, and when most women will experience labor more intensely. This is when you need to head to the birthing center or hospital. This is when contractions will be steady and will continue to increase in frequency and intensity, anywhere from three to five minutes apart. It is important to have plenty of support. This is also when you will likely start using those breathing techniques and relaxation exercises.

Pain could be centered in the thighs, lower back, or abdomen, and they can end up being intense enough that you can't talk. You may also notice a brownish or pinkish discharge, which is called a "bloody show."

This phase will usually last for three to six hours for first-timers. For women who have been induced with Pitocin, this phase will go faster, but if you choose to have an epidural, things will likely slow down. That's why you have to be a certain dilation before getting an epidural.

Don't worry if you start screaming at your partner or other people. This pain can affect people in different ways, even if you have opted for pain relief. Apologize after, but right now, it's just the pain talking.

During this phase, you will already be at the hospital or birthing center, or if you are giving birth at home, doing whatever your midwife or doula tells you to. If you are at the hospital and have opted for an epidural, you won't be able to get out of bed and will have a catheter. If you can get out of bed, you can walk around for a few minutes at a time, or march around in place. It is best to change your position if at all possible during this stage. You can also take a warm bath. You should still be drinking plenty of water and urinating periodically.

The movement helps the cervix out, and it helps to rotate the baby into place. Make sure that your partner stays actively involved during this process as well. The hospital will also monitor the baby's heartbeat.

The active labor stage can last anywhere from three to five hours. Your cervix will dilate from four centimeters to seven centimeters. Contractions will still last about 45 to 60 seconds, and you will get about a three to five-minute rest between them. They are going to be longer and stronger than the last stage.

- Transition Phase: Cervix reaches eight to ten centimeters

The mother is going to rely heavily on her support partner during this phase. This is the most challenging part, but it is the shortest. As you move through the last part of stage one before you get to the second stage, try to take things "one contraction at a time." Remind yourself of how far you have come already, and once you start feeling the urge to push, let your doctor or midwife know.

The contractions at this point are usually intense and are about three minutes apart. You can experience nausea, shakiness, and fatigue as your body works to finish dilating and effacement.

You may notice that you have a very strong urge to bear down or push along with all of the stinging in the vaginal area and pressure in the rectal area as the baby's head moves further down, but don't do it. You should wait until your doctor tells you that you can push, which won't happen until the cervix is fully dilated.

This can last from ten minutes to two hours. The best thing to do during this phase is to picture yourself in a relaxing and safe place. Breathe deep and come up with a scene that is full of details. What types of things can you see? What smells are around you? What can you hear? If you find that you can't handle the pain, you can probably still ask for pain relief. But, you may not be able to if the anesthesiologist isn't available.

Your water should have broken before this phase of stage one comes to an end. You can ask for an epidural up until you are fully dilated. It's also at the anesthesiologist's discretion. If it seems birth is imminent, they may give you an intrathecal injection of medication. The reason for this is that it takes time to set up an epidural, and the anesthesiologist needs a few minutes that are contraction free to get things into place.

### Second Stage: Pushing and Birth

Once you reach the second stage of childbirth, the cervix has fully dilated. The baby is now moving down the birth canal. This stage does not end until you give birth. Contractions are very strong and typically last for a minute. They come every three to five minutes. The contractions are pushing the baby down the birth canal, and you will likely feel intense pressure, almost like the urge to have a bowel movement.

This urge to bear down will continue, and when the cervix is completely dilated, your doctor or midwife will give you the go-ahead. Contractions won't stop, but they will come farther apart, which may give you a bit of time to rest. Some women will feel nauseous or will vomit. As you start pushing, you could become breathless and tired. This is one of the most challenging workouts that you will ever experience.

During this time, you may poop. In fact, during any part of labor, pooping is very normal. The muscles you are using to push out your baby are the exact same ones that you use to poop. Most women do poop while giving birth. It may happen multiple times or just once, normally as the baby crowns. Don't worry, though; it is all in a day's work for the people helping you.

This can last up to two hours for the first time, mom. If the baby becomes distressed, or it isn't moving through the birth canal properly, the doctor may decide to do a C-section or use forceps.

Due to the intensity of this stage, you may become irritable. There may be times when you want to be touched and talked to, and other times when you want to be left alone. It is also normal for a woman to moan or grunt once the contraction reaches its peak.

Once the baby starts to crown, you will start to feel intense pressure, possibly a stinging or burning sensation. While you are crowning, your doctor or midwife will tell you to stop pushing. This is the time where women will get an episiotomy if they need one. This is where an incision is made in the space between the vagina and rectum to widen the opening. The doctor may ask you to push more slowly or gently as the remaining part of the baby's head and the body is pushed through. With a final push, your baby is born.

During the pushing phase, it is best to get into a pushing position where gravity will work with you. Make sure that your anal area and pelvic floor are relaxed. You can also use a mirror to see how you're progressing. This can be very encouraging. Don't get upset if your baby's head emerges and then slips back in. This is a normal part of the process.

To help you understand what is going on, this is what your baby is doing at this time.

First, your baby's head will turn to one side, and the chin will automatically come to rest on the chest so that the back of the head leads the way out.

After you have fully dilated, the baby's head is front and center, and the head and torso will start to turn to face your back as it moves into the vagina.

Then the baby's head will start to crown or emerge through the vaginal opening.

After the baby's head is completely out, the head and shoulder will start to turn and face your side, which will allow the baby to move out easily.

Once you get to meet your baby, keep in mind where they have been living for the past nine months and what they just went through. Don't be surprised if they have a cone-shaped head, puffy eyes, or enlarged genitals. You may also find that they have a cheesy-type substance on them known as a vernix coating. They could also have lanugo, which is fine, downy hairs that cover their temple, forehead, back, and shoulders.

### Third Stage: Delivering the Placenta

The placenta's delivery quickly follows the amazing moment that your baby enters the world. You will probably be so amazed by your newborn that you probably won't notice this.

This is the shortest and easiest stage of labor. Once the baby has been born, and the cord has been cut, there is typically a lull. Then you will start to experience contractions once more. These are not going to be as strong as the contractions you experienced earlier. This is caused by the placenta separating from the uterine wall. You may not even notice these because you can be caught up in paying attention to your new child.

Your doctor or midwife might massage your uterus to help the placenta release. This can be uncomfortable. Once the doctor notices signs of separation, they will ask you to push again to help expel the placenta. Sometimes, the doctor may have to reach inside and pull it out. Once the placenta has been delivered, your doctor will examine it to ensure that the entire placenta is present.

All women are going to lose blood after delivery as the placenta separates from the uterus. Your body is prepared to lose this blood due to all of the blood you gained during your pregnancy.

Once the placenta has been delivered, your doctor or nurse will use their hands to push on your stomach to massage the top section of the uterus. This is called the fundus, and they are checking for firmness. They want to make sure that your uterus is staying firm, as this will prevent lots of bleeding. They may have to give you medicine to keep your uterus contracted. They will also stitch up the episiotomy or any other tears you suffered during childbirth. If you were not given an epidural, they would give you a local anesthetic before stitching you up. These stitches will dissolve.

**Labor Positions**

How do you plan on spending your labor and delivery? You might walk around a bit and then switch to squats to help push out the baby. You could lay on your side during contractions and then move to all fours once the baby is ready to be born. You could also rock on a birthing ball when the contractions are rough and then recline in your partner's arms during delivery.

It could also be a combination of all of them or just one. The great this is that it's your labor, and you get to do it your way. Getting to move into different positions during labor can ease labor pains, but it can also speed along with delivery.

You don't have just to lay down anymore. These days, moms-to-be are encouraged to labor in whatever position feels most comfortable, change up their positions if they want, and deliver in positions very different from the tradition.

This is for a good reason too. Laying on the back is one of the least effective deliver positions. In fact, any position that is aided by gravity is going to provide you with speedier results. As long as there are no high-risk conditions that may require mom to stay in bed or keep you from trying different positions, today's laboring moms, even the ones with continuous fetal monitoring and epidurals, can decide to do any deliver and labor position they want.

- Standing or Walking

Getting vertical helps gravity work with you and will allow the pelvis to open and for the baby to move down. Walking is something that you will probably do more often early on in labor than later since it is going to be harder to rush to the corridors once the contractions come more frequently. Standing is something you can do at any point. Lean against your partner or the wall for support during contractions, since it's pretty hard to stand up when you are getting squeezed below. While you can't stand and deliver, you can squat.

- Rocking

Swaying back and forth or rocking in a chair can help your pelvis to move and encourages the baby to drop further.

- Squatting

This will likely get used later on in labor or during delivery. Just like standing, squatting makes use of Newton's finest while opening up the pelvis. Your partner can be your squatting support. You can also use a birthing bar, which will keep the legs from tiring out.

- Sitting

You can sit wherever you want, and it will ease the pain of the contractions and bring gravity into play. This is also easier than squatting for long periods of time.

- Kneeling or Leaning Over

You can lean forward over a stack of pillows, chairs, or birthing ball, and this can help when you are experiencing back labor. This is because it encourages the baby to move forward, removing the pressure from your back.

- Knees and Hands

All fours is a great way to cope more comfortably if you are having back labor. This will give you the chance to do pelvic tilts while providing your partner with access to a massage and counterpressure. Some moms like to deliver in the position since it opens up the pelvis.

- Side-Lying

Better than being on your back because it doesn't compress all of those major veins, side-lying is a great option when you are too tired to sit or squat. Being on your side gives your partner better access for messages as well. Side-lying can be used as a birthing position and is great if you are experiencing a fast birth.

If you get an epidural, you can still try sitting or lying on your side. You won't be able to do anything that is going to require you to have feelings in the waist down.

Lying on your back can place a lot of pressure on your important blood vessels and can compromise blood flow to your baby, which is why you have been told not to lay flat on your back. Still, want to be in bed when you labor? Lying on your side or semi-sitting can help reduce any risk while making sure you are comfortable, and the baby is safe.

During labor, your midwife or doctor may find that some positions create changes in the baby's heart rate. If this happens, they may have you change positions.

For those looking to find out what science says about the best labor position, medical studies have found that upright positions can shorten the first stage of labor by about an hour and a half. Studies also discovered that women who spend some of the labor in an upright position had a lower risk of having to have a C-section.

Remember, it's your labor, and you can spend it in whatever position you want. You can switch up the positions when you want as well. As for delivery, whatever works well for you is the right position for you.

**C-Section**

These can be planned or unexpected. 25% of women in the US will have a C-section, so you shouldn't feel bad if you do have one. Recovery is often longer and more painful, women who deliver in this fashion can do the same thing as any other mom, and that is holding her baby and breastfeed soon after giving birth. You will be awake during it, typically, but you can't feel anything. Your partner or loved one will likely be there too. You will be able to hear things as they happen. Also, having a C-section does not prevent you from giving birth vaginally the next time.

**Partners**

The partner has a role in all of this too, and that is basically a support system. First and foremost, don't get too antsy during the first stage. You don't want to get your partner to the hospital or birthing center too early because you could be sent home. It is best to try and help her get her mind on something else, but if she asks you to stop bothering her, do that.

It's important that you paid attention to childbirth class because you are her coach. Prove to her that you are there for her and know what is going on. Try your best to be calm and focused. I know this is a big moment, but she depends on you.

Be prepared to wait, as well. Childbirth takes a long time, so have some things to distract yourself if you aren't presently needed. Your wife or girlfriend doesn't require you hovering around because your board, so read a book or something, or try to help ease her pain through a game of cards.

Try to go with the flow. Give massages, talk her through contractions, do what you have learned, but there may be a time when everything you have learned is thrown out the window. She may suddenly realize that she hates the sound of your voice or the touch of your hand. It's nothing personal; it is a pain and hormones of childbirth, but respect her demands. She may even become hostile, but this will pass.

You will also likely be helping her push, depending on what position she is in. If she is on her back, you will be on one side, the doctor on the other, supporting her under her shoulders. You will each grab a leg and bend her legs back into the right position to push.

Be prepared for the mess. If you pass out, that's okay. Lots of men do because it turns out to be messier than they thought. Other men are overcome with emotions as well. Do your best to show her your support and be a distraction when needed, and she'll love you for it later.

Lastly, enjoy the first meeting with your new son or daughter. It will be an experience like none other.

## Possible Complications

Having complications during labor and delivery is rare, but they can happen to anybody, with any doctor or practitioner, or birth setting. The majority of complications can be spotted and managed to make sure that the delivery remains safe. However, some problems can be serious and possibly life-threatening for the baby and mother.

It is perfectly normal to feel worried about the chance that something might go wrong. You could know that you have risk factors that make complications more likely. Your health care provider might tell you that certain complications can occur when you don't have an increased risk.

The following are some of the more common labor and delivery complications that you may want to talk to your doctor about so that everybody stays safe.

- Preterm Labor

This is one of the most common complications. Preterm labor is any birth that occurs before the 37th week of pregnancy. It can even start as early as 20 weeks. The CDC says that one in every ten births were preterm in 2018. Very premature babies have several challenges that they have to overcome. Even once they come home, some can experience developmental disabilities and health problems.

When you go for prenatal visits, talk to your doctor about any signs of premature labor, and find out what you can do if you experience them.

- Labor Not Progressing

Your water breaking and having contractions are typical indications of labor. Sometimes, however, this process can stop. If you started labor, but you have progressed through the stages, your doctor might have to give you medications to speed things along. Your labor could stall if:

1. Your baby stopped descending through the birth canal. This can be because the baby's head is too big to pass through the cervix, which is known as cephalopelvic disproportion.
2. Your cervix hasn't dilated.
3. Your contractions are infrequent or not strong enough.

You may have to have a C-section if things don't pick back up.

- Placenta Issues

Most placenta issues will be spotted before the baby is born, but this isn't always the case. These issues can occur after labor has started. Some problems with the placenta are more common after uterine surgery, like a C-section. Some problems could be that the placenta is covering part or all of the cervix, the placenta has grown into the uterine lining, or the placenta tears away from the wall too soon.

If this doesn't get addressed, it can cause severe blood loss that can place you at risk. Before and during labor, your health care providers will monitor you to make sure that any placenta issues are quickly treated and identified

- Umbilical Cord Problems

Issues with the umbilical cord can create issues during delivery. The cord could get wrapped around the neck of the baby, or the cord could come out before the baby. While it can be scary to think about the umbilical cord wrapped around their neck, this is usually not very dangerous.

Most of the time, it is only there briefly and is not tight enough to interrupt their breathing. If your health care professionals spot an issue with the umbilical cord, there are steps that they can take to fix the issue.

- Perineal Tearing

A tear in the tissues of the vagina and the perineal area can happen. The severity of the tear is classified using a grading system. Sometimes, it can be so bad that the provider has to fix it with stitches or in another manner. Your doctor might choose to make a cut into the tissue as you are giving birth to keep it from tearing. Whether it's an incision or tear, the wound will have to have time to recover and heal.

- Bleeding Issues

If you bleed excessively after giving birth, you will be diagnosed with a postpartum hemorrhage. There are risk factors for this. You could be at a greater risk of this complication if:

1. You have more than one child
2. You have given birth five previous times.
3. You have complications, like anemia, preeclampsia, or issues with the placenta.
4. Labor has been prolonged or had to be induced.

Talk to your doctor on how to handle bleeding during the postpartum period. Depending on the cause of the bleeding, your doctor or nurse might begin to massage the uterus or give you medication to make the bleeding stop. If the more conservative measures don't stop the problem, you might have to undergo surgery to get the placenta removed along with the uterine lining. In extreme cases, they may not be able to stop the bleeding, and the uterus could have to be taken out completely.

- Fetal Distress

Fetal distress can be caused by many different things, including umbilical cord problems, infections, induction, or medications. If your baby is having issues like shoulder dystocia, breech positioning, or perinatal asphyxia, they could show signs of distress.

External fetal monitoring will give your health care team the chance to check on the baby and see how they are handling the labor. Other tests can be performed, like internal fetal monitoring and fetal scalp pH sampling. If your baby becomes distressed and you aren't close to giving birth, they may decide to use a vacuum extractor or forceps to help with the delivery. In other cases, they may do a C-section.

The frequency of this problem is infrequent.

# CHAPTER 9: MULTIPLE BIRTHS

Multiple births only make up about three in every 100 births, but this rate is rising. There is a chance that you could wind up having more than a baby at a time. The National Center for Health Statistics has stated that the twin birth rate has gone up 70% since 1980. The rate is now 32.6 per 1000 births. The birth rate for having triplets and other multiples has risen as well, but they slowed since 1998. This could twins, triplets, or more. The actual labor process will still advance through those three stages if you can have your babies vaginal. Most of the time, especially when its three or more babies, you will likely have a scheduled C-section. Let's take a look at what it's like to have multiple babies.

## What Causes Multiple Pregnancies?

Many factors have been linked to having multiple pregnancies. These risk factors only come into play for fraternal twins. The natural causes of multiple births include:

- Race - African American women have a greater chance of having twins than other races. Native Americans and Asians have the lowest rate of having twins. White women, especially those over the age of 35, have the highest rate of having triplets or more.

- High Parity – If you have had one or more previous pregnancies, especially if those were multiples, it puts you at a higher chance of having multiples.
- Older age – Women over the age of 30 have a bigger chance of multiple conceptions. A lot of women today wait to have children until later on, and this can result in twins.
- Heredity – If you have a family history of multiple pregnancies, it raises the chance of having twins.

Other factors can raise your chances of having multiple births. These causes have an equal effect on fraternal or identical twins. These are caused by reproductive technologies and include:

- Assisted reproductive technologies – This includes IVF and other methods that can help couples have children. These make use of ovulation-stimulating medicines to cause the production of multiple eggs. They are then fertilized in the lab and placed back in the uterus to grow.
- Ovulation-Stimulating Medicines – This includes follicle-stimulating hormone and clomiphene citrate, and they help the woman

produce eggs. If they get fertilized, it can cause multiple births.

### Types of Multiple Births

You can have two types of twins. One is identical, or monozygotic, and fraternal, or dizygotic. Identical twins occur when the fertilized egg ends up splitting into two, and both halves will continue to develop into two identical children. These types of twins are genetically identical, with similar physical characteristics and the same chromosomes. They will be the same sex and will have the same eye color, hair, and blood. They are still different people and will develop separate personalities. Identical multiples can have their own amniotic sac and placenta, but most of the time, they will have separate sacs and share a placenta. Very rarely do they share one amniotic sac and one placenta.

Fraternal twins occur when the female body releases two eggs at once, and both are fertilized by two separate sperm. These children will not be any more alike than other siblings born to the same parents. They may be the same sex, or they may not. This is the more common type of twin. They can still look similar, just like regular siblings can look alike.

If you have more than two children, they are then referred to as "super twins." These babies can end up being fraternal, identical, or a combination of both.

## The Vanishing Twin

There is a chance that early on during a twin pregnancy that one of the fetuses will "disappear." This is what is known as the "vanishing twin syndrome." Even once an ultrasound has found two heart movements, spontaneous loss of one of the fetuses can still occur in up to 20% of twin pregnancies. These spontaneous losses are higher in triplet and higher-order births. There is a 40% chance of a fetal loss rate in pregnancies with three or more. If the fetus is lost during the first trimester, the remaining fetus, or fetuses, will develop like normal. Vaginal bleeding can happen.

Ultrasounds performed within the fifth week of pregnancy may not identify all fetuses. This means that you may have an "appearing twin" that is found after the fifth week. This happens about 10% of fraternal twin pregnancies and more than 80% in identical twin pregnancies. After the six to eight week mark, the ultrasound should give you an accurate assessment of how many fetuses there are.

## Diagnosing Multiple Pregnancy

Every woman is going to have different symptoms when pregnant with multiples, but some of the most common signs include:

- Fetal movements are felt in different areas of the stomach at the same time.

- Gaining more weight early on in the pregnancy.
- A bigger appetite
- More morning sickness
- The uterus grows larger than what it should be for the number of weeks during pregnancy.

When a woman suspects that she may be pregnant with more than one baby, her healthcare provider will perform some tests to make sure. Once it has been proven, she will be diagnosed with multiple fetuses. For the most part, the diagnoses take place early on in the pregnancy. The tests that may be performed include:

- Ultrasound - Through an ultrasound, they can find multiple heartbeats, which is one of the most common ways to find out you have more than one baby. They may also do a transvaginal ultrasound.
- Alpha-fetoprotein - This measures the levels of a protein that is released by the liver of the baby, which is found in the mother's blood. It will likely be higher when there is more than one fetus.
- Pregnancy blood testing - When pregnant with multiple babies, your levels of hCG will likely be higher.

**Risks With Multiple Births**

Some risks come with carrying multiple babies. These include:

- Preterm labor results in premature births

In a typical, single pregnancy it lasts 40 weeks, but twins are more often born at around 35 to 37 weeks. Over half of all twins were born before 37 weeks, and this risk of delivering prematurely increases with the number of babies. Preemies can end up having health problems. These health risks increase the earlier they are born. Because the care for these preemies is so different, they are typically taken to the neonatal intensive care unit after being born.

- Problems during pregnancy

There is a greater risk of issues like gestational diabetes, preeclampsia, placental problems, and fetal growth issues with multiple pregnancies. This is why moms pregnant with multiples will likely go to the doctor more often.

- Long-term problems

As the number of multiples increase, the more likely the child may experience developmental delays or health problems like cerebral palsy.

## Staying Healthy During Multiple Pregnancy

The best way to stay healthy while pregnant with multiples is to eat properly, get plenty of rest, and undergo regular prenatal care. You must have a health care provider that has experience with multiple births, and to do as they recommend. This is to make sure that the doctor can keep a check on any possible problems and treat them as soon as possible.

Speak with your doctor about a facility that specializes in multiple births. It is a good idea to take part in a preterm birth prevention program at the hospital and have access to a specialized NICU should you go into labor early or if one of the babies is born with health concerns.

The supplements and essential vitamins and minerals that we discussed early are important with multiple births as well, if not more important. Make sure you are getting plenty of folic acid and calcium. You are also going to want to make sure that you each more protein since you are feeding more than one baby. This will ensure that they grow correctly.

This is true for your iron intake as well. It is prevalent in multiple births to have a low red blood count. Your doctor may end up putting you on an iron supplement, as your daily requirement is going to be hard to meet through diet alone. Iron gets absorbed into the body more easily when combined with foods that have a lot of vitamin C.

Exercise is another thing you have to take into consideration. The more babies you have, the less likely you will keep up with your normal activities. Also, there are a lot of physicians who believe that a reduction in activity and increased rest will help to prolong the pregnancy and make for better outcomes. However, there has not been enough proof to show routine bed rest with multiple pregnancies can prevent preterm birth. Women who are pregnant with a high-order birth will be advised to avoid strenuous activity at some point between 20 and 24 weeks of pregnancy. This is also when they will be advised to start their maternity leave. Bed rest will help to improve uterine blood flow and can help with fetal growth problems. When on bed rest, sex is typically discouraged.

## Weight Gain

Mothers carrying multiples will need to gain more weight during their pregnancy than would be required with a single fetus. The exact amount you need to gain will depend on your pre-pregnancy weight, and how many fetuses you are pregnant with, so you will have to talk to your doctor.

The basic idea is that you would eat 300 more calories each day per fetus. This can be pretty difficult to do when your abdomen is full of babies, so it is best to have small, frequent meals throughout the day.

## Getting Ready for Delivery

Getting ready for delivery, no matter how many children you are having, can be overwhelming, but with multiplies, there is a lot more at play. This is especially true if there are already special concerns. It's important to remember that you have a network of support around you. You have capable doctors, a caring hospital staff, friends, family, and your partner there to support you.

You are likely going to be told that when carrying multiples, you should plan on giving birth earlier than the 40-week mark. This is going to lower a lot of complication risks. This means that whether or not you go into spontaneous premature labor, you will be advised as to when you should give birth.

During your pregnancy, you should discuss the options of vaginal birth and cesarean section. Even if your doctor says it is safe for you to try a vaginal delivery, things can happen where you have to have a C-section for you and your baby's safety.

You can also have other birthing attendants with you during labor and delivery. For example, you could have a midwife. We spoke about choosing a midwife over a doctor in an earlier chapter, but for multiple births, it is suggested that if you want a midwife that they work with your doctor rather alone. This is because there is a greater chance that a C-section will be required. And remember, you can also have a doula as they provided services to women during the birthing process and after delivery. Some will also go to your house after you and the babies are at home and help with household chores and infant care. Ensure you find out what services they offer and don't assume that they help in those areas.

**Delivery Process**

Labor will begin, as we discussed in the last chapter. As soon as it does, since you are having multiples, you will likely be told to go ahead and get to the hospital so that they can connect you to a fetal monitor. As mentioned in the last section, if you don't go into spontaneous labor by a certain time, you may be offered an induction to get things started, or you will just be given a C-section. The time in which doctors prefer multiples to be born, and there are no significant complications, looks something like this:

- 37 to 38 weeks for twins that have their own placenta.
- 36 to 37 weeks for twins who are sharing a placenta
- Between 32 and 33 weeks for twins who are sharing a placenta and amniotic sac.
- Thirty-five weeks if you are having triplets that have their own amniotic sacs and placentas, or if it is one baby with a separate placenta and two babies that are sharing a placenta, and all three have their own amniotic sac.

How you give birth will depend on how your pregnancy goes. When it is just twins, it will depend on the position of the first baby, where the placenta is, the growth of the babies, and how the pregnancy has gone.

If you are only having two, you may be able to have a vaginal delivery. If the baby closest to the cervix is head-down, and you don't have any other complications, your health care provider should say you are safe to have a vaginal birth. Once the first baby is born, the process will begin again for the second child. The average amount of time between the birth of the first and second child is 17 minutes. During this time, you will likely have an ultrasound to make sure that the second baby is the correct position. The pushing stage for baby number two typically goes faster because the first baby has done all of the work to get everything ready. While C-sections are prevalent for multiple births, if you only have two babies, the chances are lower. Less than half of all twins are born through a C-section. That means you have a good opportunity for birthing your babies naturally without complications. There is also the chance that your twins could be born both ways. In about 4% of all twin births, the first baby is born vaginally, and the second has to be delivered through a C-section. Again, that's very rare.

But when it comes to three or more babies, the odds of having a C-sections grows exponentially. If you undergo a C-section, you will be given a catheter, and then you will be given regional anesthesia. The most common choices are a spinal block or epidural block. This means you will be awake for the entire process, but you will be numb from the waist down. Don't worry, though, and you won't see what is going on as they put up a sheet to block your view. The babies will be born within minutes of one another. While a lot of C-sections for multiples are scheduled ahead of time, some may happen due to complications. These complications include:

- The baby is in the breech position with their feet, buttocks, or knees first, or they are lying sideways.
- You have a low-lying placenta.
- You have had problems when giving birth before.
- You have previously had a C-section.
- You have had complications during the pregnancy, or you had to be treated for problems like TTTS.
- If you are having three or more.

If the C-section has been planned and scheduled, but you go into labor early, get to the hospital immediately. You will then have an emergency C-section unless things have progressed too far or you are in very early labor, in which case a vaginal birth may be safest.

**Problems for Mom**

The risks that a present when you are having multiple babies are the same as if you were only having one, but the chances of them happening are greater. These risks include:

- Preterm labor
- Anemia
- Gestational diabetes - This type of diabetes can only occur in pregnant women, but if it is not caught and treated, it can create some serious health issues for you and the babies.
- Preeclampsia - This is a type of high blood pressure that only affects pregnant women. High blood pressure occurs when the force of your blood is too high. This can create issues during your pregnancy. Preeclampsia is only diagnosed after the 20-week mark, and it can indicate that certain organs may not be functioning properly.
- Hyperemesis gravidarum - This is a severe form of morning sickness and often requires hospitalization. In extreme cases, it can cause the placenta to dislodge from the uterus.
- Intrahepatic cholestasis of pregnancy - ICP is a condition in the liver that slows down the flow of bile, which can cause bile to build up. This bile is a fluid that helps the body to break down fats and gets rid of toxins in the body. This buildup can cause chemicals, known as

bile acids, to move into the tissues and blood. This can cause severe itching.

- Polyhydramnios - This occurs when there is too much amniotic fluid.
- Miscarriage or stillbirth
- Postpartum depression
- Postpartum hemorrhage

**How Multiples Affect the Babies**

Not only does having multiples create a higher risk of issues for mom, but it also creates a higher risk for the babies to develop problems later on in life.

- Premature birth - More than half of twins and almost all triplets and higher-order multiples will be born prematurely.
- Congenital disabilities - These are problems that are present from birth. They can affect the function or shape of a body part. They can also create problems for the baby's overall health, how the body works, and how they develop. Multiples are around twice as likely to have problems like cerebral palsy, neural tube defects, congenital heart defects, and problems with the digestive system.
- Growth problems - Multiples, mainly triplets or higher, will be smaller than singleton babies. During your prenatal checkups, your doctor will perform ultrasounds to see how the babies' are growing. If one twin becomes

much smaller than the other, they are referred to as discordant twins. These twins are more likely to develop health problems during pregnancy, as well as after birth.

- Low birthweight - This occurs if the babies weight less than five pounds eight ounces. Babies who have an LBW have a great risk of developing certain health issues, such as retinopathy of prematurity. They may also develop issues like high blood pressure later in life.
- Twin-twin transfusion syndrome - This occurs when the identical twins share a placenta, and one of them receives too much blood, while that other child does not get enough. This can be treated with laser surgery to create a seal between the babies' blood vessels. They can also perform an amniocentesis to drain off excess fluid,
- Neonatal death - This occurs when the baby dies during their first 28 days of life.

**Psychosocial Effects**

While most women who have multiple pregnancies do very well, the family might go through a lot of stress. If the mom has to be hospitalized for a prolonged stay, arrangements will have to be made for family care, home, and work.

Even when any complication has been overcome, and the babies survive without any disabilities, the effects on family life can be substantial. The impact of the multiples affects the parents, but it also affects the babies, extended family, and other siblings. Financial stress is also a common problem because of the additional costs of caring, housing, clothing, and feeding multiple children. Postpartum depression is also much more common after multiple pregnancies in the mother and father and can be long-term.

Psychological counseling and support groups can serve as a lifeline for the parents who may feel depressed or isolated. Most doctors can lead you in the right direction for mental health help.

# CHAPTER 10: BRINGING BABY HOME

Getting to bring your baby home will probably be an exhilarating moment, but it can be quickly ruined if you find you're not ready for baby. That's why it's important to make sure you have things ready before you go into labor. There's a good chance you'll start nesting before you go into labor. To make sure you are ready for your baby, let's go over some things you should make sure you have ready.

## Set Up a Place to Sleep

A lot of moms will set up a beautiful nursery for their baby, but they don't think too much about where they will sleep in their parent's rooms. The AAP says it is best to co-room with your baby for the first six months, with up to 12 months being best. This can help to reduce the baby's risk of SIDS by 50%. Sharing a room means that your baby will be sharing a room with you, but they will have their own sleeping space. The AAP says that this sleep space needs to have a flat, firm surface with tight-fitting sheets.

The sleep options for co-rooming all depend on what you want your baby to have and what adheres to the guidelines. The pack and play are great because it works with the sleep guidelines, and they can grow with the child. They typically have a weight and height limit of 35 inches and 28+ pounds. This means that they can use this up until they are a toddler. Pack and plays are also a great portable sleep space for travel.

You could also use a bassinet or Moses basket as long as they contain a flat, firm surface. The problem is that the weight limits can be anywhere from 15 to 20 pounds. This means your baby can quickly outgrow their sleeping space, and sleep space transitions can be tricky.

**Seats and Swings**

You definitely don't want to wait until the baby has arrived before you set these things up. While assembly normally isn't that hard, it is a task that is just frustrating enough that you don't need to face it when sleep deprived. You also want to have safe places to set your baby down right from the get-go. Having swings, baby bouncers, or rock and plays strategically placed in your house can make the transition back home go smoother.

If you live somewhere with more than one floor, think about having a bouncy chair on each level. Moving them between floors is a pain with a baby. It is a convenient and safe option for your baby when you are unable to hold them, or they aren't asleep.

**Diaper Station**

This is another thing you don't want to wait on. It is important to have this ready before bringing the baby home. Again, it is a good idea to have a station set up on each floor if you live somewhere with two or more floors. The central changing station will likely be in the nursery, but you can have makeshift areas around your home, so you don't have to run to the nursery every time the baby needs a diaper change. The central changing station can be on top of a dresser in the nursery, and all you need to do is place a changing table topper onto the dresser to make the space safe.

It's also a good idea to stock up on many diapers beforehand, especially if you notice a sell. Make sure you check places like Amazon or big box stores where you can buy in bulk. Baby goes through a lot of diapers. Also, you likely aren't going to need too many newborn or size one diapers. You'll be surprised at how quickly they grow. On the other hand, if you choose to use reusable diapers, make sure you have enough of them on hand, cleaned, and ready to go.

## Nursing Station

While this isn't a requirement, it is a nice thing to have and makes the transition to nursing easier. For a nursing station, you will want to have a nursing chair, a low light option, a side table, and a nursing pillow. The nursery is a good place to set up the main nursing station. Still, like with the diaper station, it's a good idea to have a mobile caddy with the supplies that you need to nurse that you can take with you downstairs, or whenever you're not going to want to have to walk to the nursery.

This may surprise you, but you will want to have some water and snacks available in the nursing station. You are going to need extra hydration to make sure you produce plenty of breast milk.

## Things You Should Learn About and Practice

There are some things you should start learning about before the baby gets here as well. One thing you will likely want to know how to do is babywearing. While you can't really practice this without having a baby, you can watch videos and learn the basics. You can also practice putting on the wrap or carrier, and you can use your partner for practice as well. Videos are much easier to follow than written instructions. With babywearing, it will ensure your baby is safe and close to you while allowing you to do things you need to do.

You should also read up on diapering. If you are planning on using cloth diapers, you will need to learn how to put them on and secure them and have diaper covers. You can also learn more about disposable diapers, such as knowing what sizes you will need.

When your baby's diaper starts leaking or experiences an explosion, it is probably a good time to change the diaper size. This, along with weight gain, will let you know when you need to change the diaper size.

## Time Management

When you don't have kids, you can do things when you want without much thought. Once you have a baby, you are going to have to work around them. This is a good time to start getting a handle on your time management. Start out by having your child in mind. Make sure you stay consistent with their routine. Children behave better when they know what to expect, and this also lets you know what to expect. Part of this is having a sleep schedule for them that you do every day.

That means they will need to take the appropriate amount of naps throughout the day and that they have a nighttime routine. Newborns will sleep most of the day. As they get older, they won't sleep as much, so set times for their naps to not sleep too much during the day. If they do, they won't sleep at night.

The schedule will also pertain to you and your partner. When they are napping, think about what you want to do during that time. This is a good time to catch up on housework, getting some work down, or relaxing. Regardless, it's important to have a consistent schedule.

### What You Have to Have Before Leaving to Have the Baby

You absolutely have to make sure that you have the car seat installed before leaving the house to have the baby. The other things we have discussed are essential as well and help to have already done, but it's not going to affect getting the baby home. If you don't have a car seat installed before giving birth, your partner will have to have it done before you can leave the hospital.

The best time to install the car seat is around the time that you would pack your hospital bag. That should be a couple of weeks before your due date.

### How to Properly Install Baby Car Seat

You have picked out the perfect car seat, and now you need to install it. You might have heard that between 75 and 96 percent of all parents do it wrong, and you want to make sure you do it right so your baby will be safe.

This is the confusing part because different car seats will have various recommendations and restrictions to install a certain car seat. Your car might have a few methods that are available to install your car seat. It doesn't really matter what way you use or the recommendations that you follow; it all begins with where.

## Location

Car seats have to be installed in the back seat. It is the safest place for children up to 13 years. Car seats shouldn't be put in the front seat due to the airbag because the airbag could cause serious injuries in a crash. The back seat will put the child farther away from the most common kind of crash, which is frontal.

Now, what is the best position to place the car seat in the back seat? The middle of the back seat is the safest place in your car, so this is the best location to install your car seat. This only works if you have one child. When you have another child, you will have to make more decisions.

## Do Some Homework

There are two things you must read before installing your car seat. The first thing is your car's owner's manual and then read the manual that came with your car seat. These give you the specifics for your car and seat. Let's say that you have chosen to put the car seat in the middle of your back seat. Your manual should tell you:

- Is your vehicle equipped with LATCH?
- If there isn't one, are you able to use a lower anchor on each side, or are you going to need to use the car's seat belt
- Some vehicles won't allow a center install.
- Your car seat manual will tell you whether or not you can use both the seat belt and the LATCH system to install your car seat... most of them won't allow it.

**Pick Your Direction**

Based on where you have selected to install your car seat, you know if you are installing it forward or rear-facing. Place the seat in your car facing the right direction for your child's age. Since this is a pregnancy book, you will be installing the car seat facing the rear.

If your car seat is a three-in-one seat or convertible, that could go either forward or rear-facing, it is going to have two different paths for the seat belt. The one for rear-facing usually runs under your baby's legs. The one for forward-facing normally runs behind your child. The right direction for your baby would be under your baby's legs.

### Angle

Just like the two different paths for the seat belt, car seats will have various angles that they have to be installed at depending on it is forward or rear-facing. Some will have an adjustable recline position. Every seat will have some type of indicator, such as a sticker that has a bubble or line for specific ranges. Some seats will have different levels that you can choose from depending on your child's age.

Make sure you have your car parked on a level surface so you can see if the indicator is right.

If it is too hard to get the right angle with just the seat's adjustability, some seats let you use a rolled towel or a pool noodle at the juncture of the seat to find the right angle for your seat.

### Getting the Seat Secured

There are three different methods you can use to make sure your seat is secure:

- Seat belt
- LATCH system if your car has it
- Both the seat belt and LATCH system - this isn't used that often. There are just a few car seats that allow this kind of installation. Make sure the manual states that it is a method that is allowed for the car seat.

Since each car seat and vehicle is different, it is important to follow all the instructions from all the manuals very carefully

- Seat Belt

Before installing your car seat in your car using this method, you have to know how to lock the seat belt. Your vehicle's manual will tell you how to do this. The most common way is by pulling the seat belt all the way out and let it go. When you release the belt, you will probably hear some ratcheting sound, and if you pull on it again, you won't be able to pull it out.

1. Put the seat belt through the right path for the direction the seat will be facing, make sure there aren't any kinks or twists, and then buckle it.
2. Look at the angle indicator to see if it is right.
3. Lock the seat belt either by using the lock off on the car seat or the seat belt mechanism. Some people will tighten the belt and then lock it. It just depends on the kind of lock you have. If the seat doesn't loosen up while you are locking it, you might have to use a locking clip to get the seat installed correctly.
4. Tighten the seat belt by getting rid of the extra webbing while putting pressure on the seat until the seat won't move more than one inch when you pull on it with your non-dominant hand. It's normal for the seat to

have some movement at the side closest to the front seat and at the top.

- LATCH

Beginning in 2003, cars were required to have two sets of LATCH systems in them. Most manufacturers placed them in the two outside seats and didn't allow you to use one anchor from each side to install a car seat in the middle. Some manufacturers placed more than two LATCH systems in the vehicle. Make sure to read your car's manual to find the position and if you can borrow one for a middle seat install. If it doesn't specifically say, NEVER do it.

Before you use your LATCH system to install your car seat, find the lower anchors in the position you are going to use. Again with a baby, you need to have them in the middle of the seat. There is normally a label or button on the seat to show you where the anchor is located.

1. Figure out which direction the LATCH clip has to be attached.
2. Be sure the LATCH strap has been routed through the right path for the seating direction. Be sure there aren't any kinks or twists.
3. Push the LATCH clips into each anchor point.
4. Look to see if it is angled correctly.
5. Tighten the strap by getting rid of the extra webbing while putting pressure on the car

seat until the seat won't move more than an inch while you are pulling with your hand that isn't dominant. It will be normal for the seat to have some movement at the side that is closest to the front seat and the top.

The LATCH system was intended to make installing a car seat easier. There could be many debates about whether or not it did or if it just added one more confusing element to the mix and a bigger chance for doing it wrong. Bot the seat belt and LATCH installations are safe up to the weight limit on the LATCH system.

The NHTSA made some changes to the LATCH system's labeling and weight limits in 2004. Basically, this means that most car seats have a combined weight of 65 pounds. They have to be labeled when you can't install it with LATCH but have to use the seat belt.

- Tethering

Car seat experts say that you need to use the tether strap for all forward-facing installations. This strap reduces the forward head movement if you get into a crash.

Find the anchor points for the tether strap in your car. Your manual should show you or your car should be labeled. Be sure it isn't a cargo hook or other kind of accessory anchor. You will pull the tether strap from the car seat over the vehicle seat's top. Clip this strap to the tether anchor point.

### More Peace of Mind

it doesn't matter what you read, and sometime it would be best to have an instructor show you. Once you have a seat installed, you can have it checked by a certified "Child Passenger Safety Technician." You should be able to find a local one by googling it. Don't take it to your local fire station or doctor unless you know they have been certified and trained.

### Dealing With Family

It's a good idea to know beforehand who you do and don't want to visit you while in the hospital, and how often. This goes for the first few weeks to months after you bring the baby home. There are a lot of people who choose not to allow extended visitors for the first two weeks after the baby comes home.

You may not want any visitors at all while in the hospital or during the first few weeks. It's a good idea, though, to be clear with family friends as to what your wishes are about visiting. Sometimes family doesn't want to follow the rules but stand your ground. If you said no visitors at all, then tell them out the door and turn them away. Their feelings might get hurt, but they will get over it. This is your time with your new baby, and it is your baby, not theirs.

If you are okay with having visitors hanging around, make sure you don't forget about feedings. Those first few weeks are crucial for successful breastfeeding, so you are going to want to feed at least every two hours if they are sleeping in somebody else's arms.

Also, you can put your visitors to work. Most people are good-natured and willing to help, but they just don't know what they should do. Don't be shy; ask them if they care to fix dinner, clean out the dishwasher, or help out in some other way.

You also need to make sure your family and friends know your social media rules. If you want to be the first person to post about your new baby's arrival, then make sure nobody takes pictures of your baby, or you tell them straight up that they are not to share anything about the baby until you do. It can be upsetting to find out a friend shared the first photos of your baby with the world.

Be blunt and upfront with family and friends. Don't assume that they won't do something because they may let you down. If you have to, give them a written set of dos and don'ts of what they can and can't do once the baby arrives. Again, it's your baby, and you have to say, other than your partner, as to what happens to them.

# CHAPTER 11: BREASTFEEDING

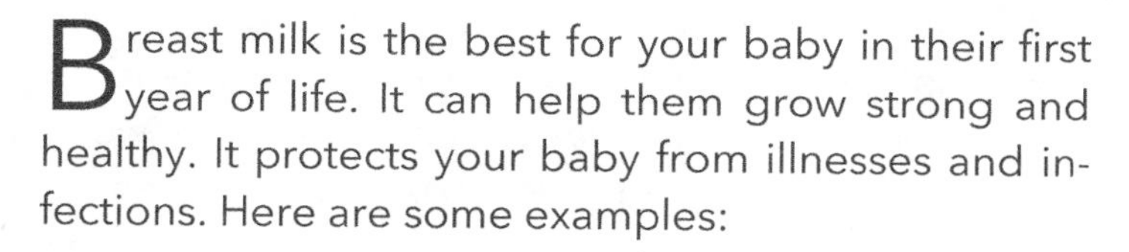

Breast milk is the best for your baby in their first year of life. It can help them grow strong and healthy. It protects your baby from illnesses and infections. Here are some examples:

- Breast milk will always be ready when your baby is hungry. You will produce more milk, the more you breastfeed.
- Breast milk will change as the baby grows, so they get exactly what they need in each stage of life. In the first few days after birth, your milk will be a sticky, thick, early type of breast milk known as colostrum. Colostrum has antibodies and nutrients that your baby needs during this time. The breast milk will change in about three days to normal breast milk.
- Breast milk is easier for the baby to digest. A baby who is breastfed might have less belly pain and gan that babies who are fed formula.
- Breastfeeding reduces your baby's risk of SIDS or sudden infant death syndrome. This is the unexplained death of a baby who is under one year of age.

- Breast milk is full of fatty acids, such as DHA, that can help your baby's eyes and brain develop.
- Breast milk is full of antibodies that protect them from several illnesses. Breastfed babies won't have as many health problems as babies who are fed formula. Breastfed babies won't have as many urinary tracts, lung, or ear infections. Later on in life, they won't develop asthma or be overweight. They also won't develop diabetes and certain cancers.
- Breast milk is full of hormones and just the right amount of fats, sugars, protein, and vitamins that help your baby develop and grow.

In the US, about 80 percent of all new moms will breastfeed their babies. About 58 percent of these will breastfeed until their babies are six months. Around 36 percent of these will breastfeed for one whole year.

**Babies Who Have Special Needs**

Babies who were born with birth defects, prematurely, or have other medical problems can be breastfed just like any other baby. Breastfeeding babies who have special needs could protect them and help them grow. Premature birth is birth before 37 weeks of pregnancy. A congenital disability is any health problem that is present at birth. They might change the function or shape of one or more body parts. They could also cause problems in the baby's overall health, how the body works, or how it develops.

If your baby has any health problems, you might need some extra help to make breastfeeding work. A lactation specialist, your doctor, or your baby's pediatrician can help your baby, and you learn how to breastfeed. A lactation specialist is a person who has had special training to help women breastfeed.

### Breastfeeding Is Good In Any Amount

It is best to feed your baby, just breast milk for the first six months. This means you don't give them solid foods, formula, water, or any other liquid, only breast milk. Any amount of breastfeeding will be good for your baby's development and health. Just breastfeeding for a short time will be good for the baby.

### Does Breastfeeding Help Mom?

Breastfeeding can help mom since:

- It helps you bond with baby.
- It might help lower your risk for ovarian cancer, breast cancer, and diabetes.
- It helps burn extra calories. This will help you get back to your pre-pregnancy weight.

- It can increase the amount of the hormone oxytocin in your body. This can help your uterus go back to its normal size. It can help stop the bleeding after you deliver your baby.

Breastfeeding can delay the return of your period. This might make it hard to know when you can start trying for the next baby. You will need to use birth control to keep you from getting pregnant until you are ready to get pregnant. Talk to your doctor about birth control that is safe for you and your baby.

### Breastfeeding Might Not Be Safe for All Babies and Moms

Breastfeeding might not be safe for your baby if:

- You use recreational drugs
- Take some types of medications
- You have specific medical problems

You could pass drugs, medicines, and infections to your baby through breast milk. Some can be extremely harmful to your baby. You need to know how to keep your breast milk healthy and safe. Speak with your doctor if you have a condition that might make breastfeeding unsafe.

## The Basics of Breastfeeding

The breastfeeding moms that you have seen make everything look so easy. They don't stop talking, they don't stop eating, they open their shirt, and that baby latches on as if breastfeeding was the most natural thing in the world. Even though the source might be natural, knowing how to nurse usually doesn't come natural at first.

It doesn't matter if your first time breastfeeding was easy, a struggle, or in between; there is a lot you can learn. The more you understand about how to position your baby (technique), how to know if your baby is getting enough milk (mechanics), and when the meal is over and when it is time for another (logistics), the more empowered and confident you will feel.

After you have gotten past the "trial-and-error" stage, and you have found the best system for you, nursing will become your most rewarding responsibility. Breastfeeding gives you and your baby a lot of benefits. It gives you both a good start on having a healthy future.

## You've Got Milk

Your breast milk will arrive in three different stages. Nature has designed each one for your baby's age. This makes it the perfect food from their birthday to their tenth day and beyond:

- Colostrum

When you give birth, your milk hasn't come in just yet. You are producing a thick substance that ranges from clear to yellow. This is known as colostrums. This is the same stuff that has been leaking out of your breasts. Colostrum is a vital blend of minerals, vitamins, and protein that can defend your baby against harmful viruses and bacteria. It could stimulate your baby to produce antibodies. It coasts the baby's intestines, protects them against digestive upset, allergies, and protects their immune system. It can also stimulate the baby's first bowel movement. It also reduces their chances of developing jaundice. You aren't going to make too much of this "liquid gold," but your baby isn't going to need more than a couple of teaspoons per feeding during their first few days. Normal feedings will help stimulate your body to make the next stage of milk in a few days.

- Transitional Milk

Next comes your transitional milk. Your breasts will begin serving this between your colostrums and the mature milk to come. This comes in between the third and fourth days. It looks like milk that has been mixed with orange juice, but it tastes a lot better. This will appear when the "first milk" comes in. It doesn't have as much protein and immunoglobulins as colostrums, but it does contain more calories, fat, and lactose. Don't worry if it seems like you are not producing a lot of milk. By day three, their tummy is about the size of a walnut.

- Mature Milk

Between day ten and two weeks after giving birth, your mature milk will come in. This will be white and thin, but it might have a slightly bluish tinge to it, too. Even though it looks like watered-down skim milk, it is packed full of nutrients and fats that your growing baby needs.

**Getting Your Baby To Latch**

At first, it might take a few tries to get your baby in the right position to get them to latch on. Just keep trying.

It is essential to know what a good latch is because an improper latching is the biggest cause of having discomfort in your breasts. Your baby's mouth needs to cover both the areola and the nipple so their lips, tongue, and mouth can massage the milk from your milk glands. Sucking on just the nipple is going to leave your baby hungry since the glands that secrete the milk aren't getting compressed. It can also make your nipples extremely sore, and they could crack. Here is how to get your latch going:

- Holding Your Baby

You need to hold your baby with them facing your breasts. The front of their body needs to face yours. You should be tummy to tummy. Their head needs to be in line with their body. Make sure their head and neck aren't crooked so they can swallow easily.

- Tickle Their Lips

Take your nipple and tickle your baby's lips with it to encourage them to open their mouth wide. They need to almost yawn. If they aren't opening their mouth, try squeezing some colostrum onto their lips.

- Baby Turn Away

If the baby turns away, begin stroking their cheek that is closest to you. Their rooting reflex will make them turn their head toward your breast.

- Bring Baby To Your Breast

Once their mouth is wide open, bring them toward your breast. Don't lean over or push your breast into their mouth. Allow your baby to take the first step. Hold onto your breast until your baby has firmly grasped your breast and is suckling.

- Will I Know The Baby Has Latched?

You will know when the baby has properly latched when the tip of their nose and their chin are touching your breast. Their lips will be flared out somewhat like a fish's lips. If their lips are tucked in, they aren't latched. Make sure your baby isn't sucking on their lower lip by pulling their lower lip down while they are nursing. Babies have a tendency to suck on anything.

- Look for Suckling

Watch to see if the baby begins suckling. Once they have, you've done it. They are extracting colostrum or milk from your breasts. They aren't just gumming or sucking your nipple. If your baby is suckling, you will see a steady and strong "suck-swallow-breathe" pattern. You will notice a rhythmic motion in their ear, jaw, and cheek. When your milk comes in, listen for sounds of gulping or swallowing. You will know if they are latched properly, as you will hear clicking sounds.

- Baby Can't Latch On Properly

Gently break the suction by carefully pressing a clean finger against the corner of their mouth. You could also press on your breast near their mouth. Start tickling their lips with your nipple again and allow them to properly latch on again with your areola and nipple in their mouth.

**How Long Should You Allow Them to Eat**

You might have heard that short feedings prevent cracking and soreness. This normally doesn't come from feeding too long but from getting into the wrong position. Rather than setting time limits on your feedings, allow your baby to take their time and expect the feedings to belong.

- Feeding Normally Last Between 20 and 30 Minutes

Remember, that is the average. Your baby might take more or less, and they might want to feed longer at first and during any growth spurts.

- Completely Drain One Breast

At least one breast needs to be well-drained at every feeding. This is actually more important than having the baby feed from both breasts because the hindmilk (the last of the mature milk that your baby gets) will be richer in calories and fats. Don't stop them from feeding too early. Wait until they seem like they are ready to stop with the first breast and then offer them the next. If they aren't interested in the other breast, begin with this one the next time.

- Baby Will Tell You When They Are Done

You need to end their feeding by waiting until your baby lets go of your nipple. If they don't, you can end it when the "suck-swallow" pattern slows down to about four sucks to one swallow. Most of the time, your baby will fall asleep by the time they get to the end of the first breast, and they will either wake up to nurse from the next, or they will sleep until their next feeding. Remember to unlatch them by gently pressing against the corner of their mouth with your finger or press against the side of the breast near their mouth.

**How Often Should You Breastfeed**

Feeding a baby when they are hungry instead of on a schedule is best for having success at breastfeeding. Since babies aren't born being hungry, their appetite normally increases around day three. There probably isn't going to be much demand at first. This means you have to initiate or push them at first.

Newborns need to have between eight and 12 feedings in a 24-hour timeframe, even if the demand isn't there yet. Break it down, and you should be feeding baby every two or three hours, day and night. You will begin counting from the start of each feeding.

Feeding patterns are going to be different for every baby, but so might need to nurse less or more frequently. If you have an impatient or hungrier infant, you might not go more than one hour between your feedings. A baby that is easily satisfied might go between three and four hours. If you feel as if you are nursing all the time, don't worry, this will be temporary. As your supply of milk increases and your baby gets older, the breaks in between feeding will get longer.

Don't be surprised or worried if your friends who formula-fed their babies tell you that their baby didn't eat as often. Breast milk can be digested easier than formula, and this lets nursing babies tummies empty out faster, and they will want to be fed sooner.

### How to Know If Baby Is Hungry

The best way to get the correct balance when breastfeeding is to nurse anytime your baby seems to be hungry. Don't wait until they are crying uncontrollably; by this time, your baby might be too hungry. They may be small, but they will make their needs known by:

- Smacking their lips
- They are sucking on their tongue or lips. This might look like they are sticking their tongue out at you.
- Rooting, they will open their mouths and turn their head to the side with their mouth open, trying to find food.
- Opening their mouth wide

- Sucking on the hand, your arm, or your shirt
- Nuzzling your breasts
- If they do cry, it is normally a low-pitched, short wail that will rise and fall.

**Breastfeeding Positions**

While you are in the hospital or birthing center, they will probably teach you the basic cradle hold. With some "trial-and-error," you might find other positions that work better for you. Here are some of the most popular breastfeeding positions:

- "Biological Nurturing" or Laid-Back Position

For this position, you will lean back on pillows to support your head, neck, and back. You won't be lying flat down but in a semi-reclined position. Put the baby on you with their tummy against yours. They will be lying on your chest in any direction that works for both of you. Place the baby's cheek against your breast. Their weight gets supported by your body. The ideas behind this position are taking advantage of gravity and allowing your baby to find your nipple. You can still hold your breast and point it toward them to encourage them to latch. This is a great position for babies who have sensitive tummies, are gassy, or who spit up a lot. It leaves your hands free to caress and cuddle your baby.

- Side-Lying

This is a good position if you are nursing in the wee hours of the morning. Lie on your side with your head supported by a pillow. Baby is facing you, of course, their head close to your nipple. You can use your hand that isn't on the side that you are lying on to cup your breast if needed. You could place a small pillow behind your baby's back to help support them.

- Football Hold

In this position, your baby's legs will be tucked under your arm on the same side as the breast that you are nursing from. Hold the baby with that arm supported on a pillow to lift them up. You can sue your other hand to hold your breast if needed.

- Crossover Hold

To get into this position, you will hold your baby's head with the hand on the opposite breast that you will be nursing from. If you are nursing from your right breast, hold their head with your left hand. Use your free hand to cup the breast if you need to.

- Cradle Hold

You will position your baby, so their head is resting in the bend of your elbow on the arm on the side that you will be breastfeeding from. The same hand will be supporting the baby's body. Hold your breast with the other hand and compress it gently, so your nipple is pointing toward the baby's nose. Encourage them to latch onto your nipple to begin feeding.

**How to Know If Baby Is Eating Well**

Many new moms who are first-time breastfeeders worry that their baby isn't eating enough. You can't calibrate your breast to know how much milk they have in them or how much is being taken out. If you are worried, some indicators can help you check to make sure they are getting full:

- Weight

Babies need to gain weight each week from their second week onward steadily. Around four to seven ounces each week is normal for newborns, even though their weight will vary according to age and other factors. Their pediatrician will tell you if your baby's growth is on track.

- Dirty Diapers

I know this sounds a bit odd but count your baby's diapers. After about three to four days, your baby should be filling up between six and 12 diapers with very pale yellow or clear urine and about three or four yellowy, soft bowel movements daily. For the first few weeks, it is a good idea to write down how often your baby feeds, and when you change their diaper. You can bring this with you to their doctor visits.

- Disposition

If your baby seems content and happy after you feed them, then they are probably one satisfied little customer, and they are getting all the milk they need. If they are sucking on the fingers, fussing, or crying, they are probably still hungry. These can be signs of colic or gassiness, too.

**Storing Breast Milk**

Knowing how to store and prepare your breast milk for healthy babies all depend on some factors: where you will store it, the kind of breast milk, and at what temperature. If this is a bit hard for you to remember, just think about the "rule of fours." For breast milk that has just been pumped, you can give leave it at room temperature for four hours or up to four days in the refrigerator.

To keep your breast milk from being wasted, store in small batches. It is recommended for about two to four ounces. Any breast milk that remains in the bottle after your baby has eaten needs to be consumed within two hours or if refrigerated at their next feeding.

You can always thaw a bottle if needed, and you do have some options in kinds of containers you can use:

- Breast milk storage bags. Never use disposable bottle liners or other plastic bags to store your breast milk. These are too tink and could start leaking. Plus, there is a higher fat loss when milk gets stored in polyethylene bags.
- Sterile BPA-free plastic or glass bottles that have lids the fit tight. Don't use containers that have a recycling number of three or seven as these might contain BPA.

Breast pumps, along with all the supplies you need to help you with lactation, qualify as tax-deductible. The IRS does not give a specific list of items that they approve other than the pump; if the product gets used for any medical reason, even the cream for cracked nipples, it will qualify as a tax-deductible item. Keep track of everything you spend and look at your insurance policy. Some insurance covers the cost of breastfeeding supplies like breast pumps and storage bags.

### How Long to Keep Breast Milk In the Refrigerator?

Breast milk will separate into a creamy top layer and the milk layer underneath when it gets stored. It will look a bit funky, but it is safe and normal to swirl together before you feed it to your baby.

How long you can keep the milk in the refrigerator depends on a few things:

- Breast milk that has just been pumped can be put in the back of the refrigerator at a temperature of 39 degrees for no longer than four days. Try not to forget you put it there.
- Previously frozen milk that has been thawed can only be in the fridge for 24 hours before you get rid of it. Only take out of the freezer what you know your baby will consume in one day. You CAN'T refreeze breast milk after it has been thawed.
- If your baby doesn't consume all of the milk during a feeding, you need to use it in two hours or put it in the fridge to be eaten at the next feeding.

When you warm breast milk from the refrigerator, put the bottle into a bowl of warm water, or hold it under warm running water. NEVER microwave breast milk.

**How Long to Keep Breast Milk In the Freezer?**

You can store your breast milk in the freezer attached to your refrigerator at zero degrees for nine months. If you have a deep or chest freezer at -4 degrees, you can store the milk for one year.

The earlier you use the milk, the better since long storage could diminish the vitamin C content in the milk. The temperature in the freezer needs to stay at zero or lower. It is best to keep it in the back or farthest away from the door where the temperature remains consistent.

### How to Know If the Breast Milk Is Still Good

If you know what spoiled milk smells like, they will know what spoiled breast milk will smell like. If you still aren't sure, just taste it. If it tastes sour, then it is bad, and you should pour it out.

There is one more trick. Watch how the breast milk moves. If the breast milk is still good, it will mix together easily when you gently swirl it around in the bottle. If it doesn't or has chunks floating in it, get rid of it.

Remember that breast milk stored in a freezer should be used in six months for the best quality of milk, but you can keep it for one year.

# CHAPTER 12: DEALING WITH SPECIAL CONCERNS

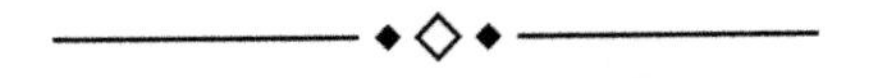

It could be a bit nerve-wracking when you are a new parent, and that is entirely understandable. Some new parents don't know what they should expect within the first year after their baby is born. Various types of illnesses will strike at some point because infants are very vulnerable to disease or infections than older children.

The good news is that most of these illnesses are very common and easy to treat without having to take them to the doctor. But, infants could contract more serious problems that will require a doctor's attention. The following common illnesses could help you identify which condition needs a doctor and when you should call.

## Common Health Problems in Infants and Newborns

Babies are very vulnerable right after birth, and while they are making the transition from the safety of the mother's womb into this world. This is the time when they learn how to feed, breathe, and more. This is also the time when their liver, kidneys, brain, heart, lungs, etc. learn to coordinate. If they feel any kind of discomfort, the only way they can talk to you is through crying. With you being the parent, you have to try to understand what could be troubling your baby and talk to their doctor as quickly as possible.

- Injuries At Birth

There might be times when a baby suffers a physical injury during birth. This could happen if the labor were very difficult or long or if the baby was quite large. Even though newborns normally recover reasonably quickly from some injuries, others might last longer. Sometimes the damage might be a broken collarbone. This will heal as long as the arm is kept motionless. Once a couple of weeks has passed, there may be a small lump that forms at the fracture, but this is a good thing. It shows that the new bone has started to form and mend the broken one.

Muscle weakness can occur when stretching or pressure is placed on the nerves attached to various muscles. The muscles can end up being weakened on a single side of the arm, face, or shoulder. This normally goes back to normal after a few weeks. Just ask their pediatrician to show you how you can hold them to help them heal and to nurse them.

- Marks From Forceps

If forceps were used to help during the birth of your baby, they might leave behind some red marks or even some scrapes on the head and face of the baby where the metal touched them. This normally disappears in a couple of days. At times, a flat but firm lump will develop in this area due to the slight damage to all of the tissues located under their skin. This, once again, will fade after a few months.

- Excessive Crying

All babies are going to cry and, most of the time, for no reason whatsoever. If you know that your baby has a clean diaper, is warm, has been burped and fed, the next best thing to try is to hold them as you sing or talk to them until they calm down. You can't "spoil" the baby by giving them attention. If this does not help calm the baby down, then try swaddling them in a blanket.

You are going to start getting more use to your baby's patterns of crying. If they ever sound peculiar, like they are in pain, or it lasts for a long time, it might mean there is an underlying medical problem. Call their pediatrician and ask them what you should do.

- Constipation

It isn't uncommon for a baby to have irregular bowel movements within their first year of life, especially when introducing new foods into their diet. Once babies start eating solid foods, they might experience some constipation and won't be able to pass a solid stool. Several home remedies can help, and one of them is dietary changes.

If your baby has chronic constipation, their doctor might prescribe them some suppositories, or they might want to do some testing for another medical problem. If you ever see blood in your baby's diaper, call their doctor immediately.

- Diarrhea

This is the complete opposite of constipation. Babies who have diarrhea will have bowel movements that are too watery and too frequent. Diarrhea could be caused by medication, bacterial infection, food allergy, and it might cause your baby to become dehydrated. Just like constipation, a stool that is bloody requires a doctor's attention immediately. Some other signs that a doctor's attention is needed include dry eyes, weight loss, vomiting, and fever.

- Jaundice

This is a common condition for many infants and newborns. It happens when there is too much bilirubin in the baby's blood. This causes the skin to have a yellow pigmentation. This is fairly common because many babies are born with neonatal jaundice. This happens since the baby's liver isn't mature enough to flush out the extra bilirubin that is in the blood. While most babies will have a bit of jaundice, it becomes a problem if their levels of bilirubin get too high. Even though jaundice is treatable like when the bilirubin levels get too high and it doesn't get treated right, it could lead to brain or nervous system damage. This why it is important that this gets checked and treat accurately. Jaundice is usually more common in breastfed babies and usually the ones who don't nurse well. Breastfeeding moms need to make sure that the nurse eight to 12 times during the day. This is going to help keep their milk production up and to lower the bilirubin levels.

Jaundice is most commonly noticed on the face, and then it will move into the chest and abdomen. After that, it will spread into the legs and arms. You might even notice the whites of their eyes are a bit yellow, too. Their doctor will check for jaundice, and if they think that there is any, they might have a blood or skin test done to give a proper diagnosis. If jaundice appears on the skin before the baby is 24 hours old, the doctor will need to do a bilirubin test to get an accurate diagnose. Once the baby reaches three to five days old, babies will have to have a doctor's appointment because this is when the bilirubin levels will reach their highest. This is why if the baby is discharged from the hospital before they reached three days old, they have to be seen by a pediatrician in two days. Some babies will have to be seen sooner, including:

- Babies who have a sibling or parent who has high levels of bilirubin and had to take treatment for it
- Babies with a lot of bleeding and bruising under their scalp that was associated with their birth
- Babies who aren't breastfeeding well
- Babies who had jaundice appear within 24 hours after birth
- Babies who were born more than two weeks early
- Babies who had high levels of bilirubin before they left the hospital

If their doctor figures out that jaundice are present in your baby and they need to be treated, their bilirubin levels could be reduced by putting the baby under special light when they aren't dressed. This can be done at home or in the hospital. Their eyes will be covered to protect them from light therapy. This treatment could prevent all the harmful effects that jaundice might bring. In babies who are breastfed, jaundice might last for a couple of weeks. In babies who are fed formula, jaundice will go away in a few weeks.

- Abdominal Distension

This can happen in healthy babies. The main cause of abdominal distension is swallowing too much air. You being the parent, have to watch your baby's belly. Newborns will have soft and protruding bellies. If your baby's tummy looks swollen and feels hard, any time you touch it, it might be due to constipation or gas. As their bodies begin adjusting to feedings, the problem should go away by itself. But, if you see a bluish tinge on their skin, the problem persists, they haven't had a bowel movement in a couple of days, they are vomiting, and there is a lot of distension to their stomach, it might mean there is an underlying problem with their internal organs.

- Skin Conditions

Specific issues such as cradle cap and diaper rash are common skin problems that can be painful for your baby. They might get diaper rash if they have worn a dirty or wet diaper for too long. It could also be an allergic reaction to the dyes in the diaper. Changing your baby's diaper and using a quality diaper rash cream can clear it up in no time. If your baby develops cradle cap, it might be due to excess oil production in the skin surrounding the hair follicles. The symptoms of cradle cap will be "scales" on their scalp. Washing their hair with a mild shampoo daily can loosen up and get rid of the "scales." This condition should clear up in a couple of months; if it doesn't, call their doctor.

- Ear Infections

If your baby begins pulling or rubbing at their ears, they don't want to lie down, and they are crying more than normal, it might be possible that they have an ear infection. Ear infections happen when germy fluid gets accumulated in the ear. This begins pressing on the eardrum and can cause a lot of discomfort for your baby. Ear infections do require a doctor's attention because they could lead to hearing loss if left untreated. If you catch the infection early enough, your doctor can give your baby an antibiotic that will heal it.

- Oral Thrush

This is a yeast infection that happens in a baby's mouth. This is also known as oral candidiasis and is very common in babies. Symptoms of this will be white lesions on the inner cheek or tongue. If you think your baby has this, call your doctor to see if it is serious enough for anti-fungal medication.

- Fever

Fever is one indication that your body is trying to fight off some kind of infection. But a high fever over 101 degrees that won't go away with fever reducers in babies could cause brain damage and seizures. If your baby had a high fever, you need to take them to the doctor as soon as you can to get some medication.

- Apnea and Bluish Skin

Newborns can sometimes have feet and hands that are a bit bluish. This blue color will fade with time as their circulation improves throughout their body. If their feet and hands turn blue when they are cold, they should turn back to pink when they get warm. Their lips, tongue, and face might turn blue when they are crying hard, but when they calm down, their color should come back to normal. If you see a bluish tinge around the baby's mouth and it stays there for a long time, and you notice they are having problems breathing, this might mean your baby's lungs and heart aren't functioning right. Your baby might have apnea if their breathing stops between 15 and 20 seconds, and their skin is slightly blue. They might have a heart problem that needs medical treatment immediately.

- Vomiting

There are going to be times when your baby is going to spit up the milk that you feed them. This is common with babies. This is why you need to burp your baby to keep them from throwing up. After you feed your baby, if they throw up the milk and you see a greenish color in their vomit, and they continue to vomit, it could cause serious problems. Babies can get dehydrated extremely quickly, and medical help is needed. Breast milk and lactose intolerance is relatively common and needs to be monitored. Frequent spitting up and vomiting of milk might be due to digestive problems or an infection.

- Respiratory Distress

It can take a baby a few hours after they are born to create a regular breathing pattern, but they shouldn't have any problems after that. If they seem to be breathing unusually, it is usually from a blockage in their nasal passages. Using saline nasal drops, followed by using a bulb syringe, might be all you need to fix the problem. You can find both of these in most pharmacies.

If your baby begins showing any of the following warning signs, call your pediatrician immediately:

- Blue skin that won't go away
- Grunting while trying to breathe
- Flaring their nostrils

- Retractions: This is when the muscles between their ribs suck in when they breathe, so their ribs are sticking out
- Breathing fast: This would be more than 60 breaths per minute. Just remember that babies do breathe faster than adults

- Flu and Colds

Babies have delicate immune systems, and this means that they are more likely to contract illnesses from the people around them. Many babies will have many colds during their first year, which comes with a runny nose, sneezing, and coughing.

It is a good idea to talk to their doctor if your baby is showing signs of the flu or cold, as these illnesses, even though mild, could easily develop into pneumonia. Their doctor might recommend an OTC cold medicine that is safe for your baby. You shouldn't give your child any type of medicine without talking to their doctor first.

- Sleepiness and Lethargy

All babies spend a lot of time sleeping. As long as they wake up every couple of hours, they eat well, they seem content, and they stay alert for part of their day, it is normal for them to sleep. If they aren't alert a lot, don't wake up on their own to be fed, or they don't seem interested in eating or act too tired to eat, you need to talk to their pediatrician. This lethargy, especially if it is sudden, might be a symptom of an illness.

- Coughing

If your baby coughs while they are getting fed, the milk might be flowing too fast. Persistent gagging and coughing while feeding might indicate a problem with their digestive system or lungs. Coughing during the night constantly might indicate respiratory problems or whooping cough. If your baby coughs while they are being fed, or during the night, you need to take them to their doctor as soon as you can.

- Anemia

Babies who are born to anemic mothers will be anemic, too. Anemia is a condition where the red blood cells are less than normal for the child's age. Anemia is a lack of hemoglobin. This shows that the amount of oxygen in the blood is lower, and the blood is very thick. Medical intervention is needed because if left untreated, it could result in death.

- Colic

If your baby is crying for no reason, especially during the evenings, this is normally called colic. The true cause of colic isn't known, but some of the theories behind it suggest it could be caused by overstimulation of sound or light, hormones causing stomach pain, gas, or their digestive system is growing. Colic might also be by gastroesophageal reflux. This is when the contents of the stomach that are very acidic come back up into the esophagus. Colic could start at about two weeks if the baby were full-term, and it should go away by the time the baby gets to three months. If this condition persists, it might be due to an intolerance to their formula, milk, or other conditions. It would be best to talk with their doctor to get a diagnosis.

If your baby is continuously crying and they are over the age of three months, it is time to call their doctor. Their doctor might recommend smaller but frequent feedings, a different formula, or particular medications.

Most diseases and problems with babies typically resolve by themselves with some time as baby's bodies get stronger, and they learn how to cope. Parents do need to be careful. Take the baby for their normal checkups to their pediatrician. Keep them clean and keep a clear and calm mind. If your baby is experiencing any discomfort, please don't hesitate to call your doctor. But, above all, enjoy the arrival and this adjustment phase with your bundle of joy. Not every sneeze or cough is going to be something serious. A baby who is sick can cause new moms to worry but having a pediatrician that you trust and who is just a phone call away is a great comfort.

## Health Problems That Can Affect New Moms

After you have a baby, you are going to focus more on your baby than you will on yourself. Even though your baby's development will be marvelous, you might experience some changes, too. Your health problems are just as important as your baby's. Most people only focus on preparing for their pregnancy and ways to be healthy during pregnancy, but they don't know how to take care of themselves after they give birth.

Here are some common health problems you can expect:

- Breast Pain

If your breasts get painful, hard, lumpy, or swollen, they are engorged. This happens as the body tries to figure out the amount of milk it needs to produce while getting its milk supply.

You can apply warm compresses before you breastfeed to help your milk flow easier. You can take acetaminophen and use ice packs between feedings. Breastfeeding could be uncomfortable and painful for some women but hang in there.

You might have heard that nursing comes naturally. But the truth is that for many new moms, that isn't true. It might feel natural after several weeks, but it will take some practice and hard work to get it right.

Moms feel a lot of pressure from the family, friends, and doctors to nurse their babies. Even though the whole medical community recommends you breastfeed for the benefits that it gives both child and mother, it is best to think about the bottle-versus-breast debate. The most important thing to remember is that the feedings are comfortable for both your baby and you. Basically, this means that if you feel frustrated and tense when you try to nurse your baby, you are doing anyone any favors.

If you experience pain while breastfeeding, you could meet with a lactation specialist who can help your baby latch on properly to eliminate the pain. If you have a close friend who breastfed their baby, you can also ask them to watch you see if you are doing anything wrong. They might have some suggestions that will make things easier for you. It might help just knowing that you are doing everything correctly, and it will get easier. Make a goal of sticking with it for one month because it could take that long just to get the positioning and timing down. If you are still frustrated and things aren't going well, you can switch to using formula.

- Vaginal Pain

Women are generally aware of the pain they are going to experience during childbirth; what most don't realize is all the pain they will have after. With vaginal deliveries, it all depends on if the delivery went smoothly, and if an episiotomy or lacerations was needed and repaired. If you do have some pain, try a pain-relieving spray or ice.

Those who had to have a C-section might experience a bit of pain around the incision. You will likely get prescription pain medication that you will have for around two weeks. After that, ibuprofen or Tylenol should work.

- Infection

Childbirth can be tough on the body. Other than infection at the C-section site or possibly a tear in the perineum, you could get an infection in the kidneys, bladder, or uterus.

These infections are not that common unless there is a problem with delivery, such as prolonged rupture of membranes or prolonged labor. You just need to watch for increased pain or fever. If any of these symptoms come up, it might be an infection that can be treated with antibiotics.

- Pelvic Organ Prolapse

Pregnancy can weaken the pelvic floor, and childbirth weakens it even further. In some women, this could cause a prolapse. A prolapsed happens when the bowels, uterus, or bladder protrudes into the vagina. This condition will lessen with rest. This means you shouldn't pick up anything heavier than your baby.

While some women will experience a prolapsed during the postpartum time, it is going to get better, but there is still a slight chance that it can come back after a woman goes through menopause. Don't worry about it and just keep it to yourself. There is some treatment available.

- Incontinence

You are going to need to remember every public bathroom that you mapped out during your pregnancy. Being incontinent is common during the first six months after delivery. Building up your pelvic floor muscles could help your incontinence.

- Being Exhausted

New moms are going to be tired, and that is completely understandable. The first two or three months are going to be a complete blur just because of your baby's feeding schedule. It is normal for the first two weeks to cry easily or feel moody because of exhaustion and not enough sleep. Try to get prepared before the baby comes by making sure you have all the things you need at home.

Use your support system to help you with nighttime feedings so you can get a couple of nights' sleep. If your moodiness persists or gets worse and you feel like you are going into an uncontrollable sadness, you feel worthless, or you want to sleep all the time, ask your doctor about postpartum depression. There is a separate section about postpartum depression below.

- You Have To Do Everything Right

Mothers are under tremendous pressure. You shouldn't live in sweat, their children have to be happy, or your house has to be excessively clean. Trying to be perfect is going to make you crazy. Just try to be "good enough." This means giving your baby a loving and safe environment. You need to accept the fact that you are going to make mistakes and your house is going to be messy, and you might have to go a week without getting a shower. Rejecting this "perfect mother" myth means you have to resist the urge to micromanage your day. New moms think they have to be singing or talking to their baby all day, or they have to pick them up every time they cry. Babies need their downtime, too. They can be content just lying there staring at the fan.

Never feel guilty about putting your baby in their swing or bouncy seat for a short time while you take a shower, eat lunch, or just relax for a few minutes. Accept the fact that babies are going to cry. Don't take their crying as a sign that you are failing as a mother if you can't get them to stop crying immediately.

You also need to ignore all the criticism that you may get from friends, strangers, and family about how you are doing. Some people just like to run their mouth about things by saying that you are going to spoil your baby by simply holding them when they cry or that you didn't dress them warmly enough when you took them outside. Just thank them for their tips and just do what feels right for you.

- What About Your Job

For some women, making the decision about going back to work after your baby is born is really a no-brainer. Your family might need your paycheck to survive. But for moms who have a choice about whether they want to be a stay-at-home mom or a working mom, this decision can be agonizing. There are a lot who will wonder if they made the best decision. When you are home all day alone with your baby, all by yourself can make you feel isolated. Some stay-at-home moms may discover that they miss their old work, co-workers, and the community. Working moms usually feel guilty that they aren't with their children all the time.

Find moms who are struggling with these same problems. Give your choice a time limit of one year. Just because you made one decision doesn't mean you can't change your mind later. Ask yourself: "What am I going to do this year?" You can make the decisions that it's not working for you and make a change. Try talking to your employer about getting a flexible schedule or pick up a part-time job that will provide you what you are looking for.

- You Think You Are Fat

When you turn on your television or walk by a newsstand, you see millions of pictures of celebrity moms who are skinnier than ever. New moms think that they are going to be back in the pre-baby clothing just like that after giving birth. If you don't have a personal trainer and a nanny, it might take some time for your body to seem like yours again. Mothers who lose the weight quickly are the minority. Many women take a year to get back into their pre-baby clothes.

Even the ones who shed the pounds fairly fast might be shocked to find their body has morphed in another way. Childbirth will come with some war wounds. Suddenly,, you notice that your hips are wider, you have varicose veins, and you are losing hair. This might be a sign that you have postpartum depression.

You have to remember that all of those extra pounds are serving an important role. This is storing fat and energy that you are going to need for breastfeeding. While getting a bit of exercise is good, don't stay super focused on losing that weight. Put your baby in a stroller and take a walk. This is a good way to exercise and to destress. Give your partner some credit. They likely won't even take notice of those stretch marks or pounds. They just want the two of you to reconnect.

- You Hate Your Partner

Fine, hate might be a powerful word. Some new moms believe that having a baby is going to bring them closer to their partner, but are surprised to find that they are screaming at them more. You might even think about getting a divorce thousands of times during your baby's first year. This is completely normal. Adjusting to this new role adds a lot of stress to the most vital relationships. New moms might feel their partner doesn't understand what they are going through all day long. They might resent having to all the household chores plus taking care of the baby that they thought was going to be split evenly. Men might feel more pressure to succeed at work so they can financially provide for their families. It isn't any wonder that the mood in the house is usually anything but nice and romantic.

First, you have to realize that your partner is doing the best they can. Realize that taking care of a child is hard, and it is going to stress out your relationship for some time. The best thing you can do is talk about the things that are bothering you. Let your partner know you need them because they can't read minds. If you really feel like you have been doing all the cooking and cleaning, don't get angry about it. Sit them down and make a list of what each one of you could do. At times, having your partner take over a night feeding so you can get some sleep, or ask them to do the laundry for a few days, can make a world of difference.

There are going to be a lot of new life changes and health problems that can impact new moms after they give birth, but knowing what to expect will go a long way to prepare your body and mind. This is an exciting time for your family. Be sure you have all the support you need so you can just focus on cherishing each moment with your baby.

### Postpartum Depression

Postpartum depressions is a mixture of behavioral, emotional, and physical changes that happen in some women after giving birth. This is a form of major depression that could start about four weeks after the birth of their child. Being diagnosed with postpartum depression is based not just on the length of time between delivery and onset of depression symptoms, but on how severe the depression is.

Postpartum depression has been linked to psychological, social, and chemical changes that can happen after having a baby. It is a range of emotional and physical changes that most new moms experience. Postpartum depressions can be treated with counseling and medication.

Chemical changes involve the quick drop in hormones after giving birth. The link between depression and this drop in hormones isn't clear. What they do know is the levels of progesterone and estrogen increase A LOT during pregnancy. Then once they give birth, they drop just as sharply. By the third day after giving birth, these hormone levels are back to where they were before you were pregnant.

Other than these chemical changes, the psychological and social changes of having a baby make an even greater risk of depression. Many new moms will experience what most people call the "baby blues" after giving birth. Around one in every ten moms will develop a long-lasting and more severe depression after giving birth. Around one in every 1000 women will develop a severe condition known as postpartum psychosis.

- Signs and Symptoms

Some of the symptoms of postpartum depress can be hard to see. Most women will have these symptoms:

- o Frequent mood changes
- o Decreased libido
- o Excessive fatigue
- o Changes in appetite
- o Problems sleeping

With postpartum depression, these could be accompanied by symptoms of some major depression that aren't typical after giving birth, and they might include:

- You think about hurting others
- You think about suicide
- You feel helpless, hopeless, and worthless
- You don't feel pleasure
- You are always in a depressed mood

New symptoms of OCD don't usually happen during the postpartum period. These obsessions are typically related to worrying about your baby's health. You might also have some irrational fears about hurting your baby. Panic disorders might again happen. You could have depression, and these conditions together.

Untreated postpartum depression could be dangerous for new moms and their babies. New moms need to get professional help if:

- You are feeling very panicked, scared, or anxious all the time
- You have thoughts of hurting your baby or yourself
- You can't cope with daily problems
- You can't function normally
- Your symptoms last longer than two weeks

- Treatment for Postpartum Depression

Postpartum depression gets treated differently depending on the severity and type of symptoms. Treatment options could include antidepressant or anti-anxiety medication, finding a support group for education and emotional support, and psychotherapy. For severe cases, intravenous infusions of a new medicine known as brexanolone might be prescribed.

If you develop postpartum psychosis, drugs that are used to treat psychosis might be added. Hospital admission might be needed.

If you breastfeed your baby, don't just think that you can't take medicine for psychosis, anxiety, or depression. Speak to your doctor. Women can take medications while breastfeeding as long as they are the supervision of a doctor. This is a decision that has to be made between your doctor, your partner, and yourself.

# CHAPTER 13: 10 IMPORTANT POINTS ABOUT PREGNANCY

You can find information about pregnancy everywhere. During your first prenatal visit, your doctor probably gave you a bag full of pamphlets along with other things to help you understand what your body will be going through. Plus, you have read this book up until this point. In spite of all the information you have been given so far, there are some essential points about pregnancy that you need to know.

### Constipation, Hemorrhoids, and Varicose Veins

Varicose veins are caused by blood pooling in enlarged veins that were created by all of the extra hormones during pregnancy. These are generally located around the genital area and legs. They normally go away once you have given birth. There are some things that you can do to prevent them:

- Keep your feet raised when sitting
- Wear support hose
- Wear clothes that fit you loosely
- Try not to sit or stand for too long

Hemorrhoids are varicose veins located in the rectum. These are very common during pregnancy, also. The amount of blood flowing through your body has increased, and your uterus is sitting heavy on the pelvis. Hemorrhoids can be extremely painful; they could sting, itch, or bleed after or during a bowel movement.

Another common pregnancy problem is constipation. This happens due to the pregnancy hormones slowing down the digestive process. During the last few months of pregnancy, the uterus could push up against the large intestines, making it more difficult to have a bowel movement. Constipation can make hemorrhoids worse due to you having to strain to use the bathroom, making the veins of the rectum larger.

The best thing to do for these problems is to make sure they don't happen in the first place. Eating a diet of fiber-rich foods, drinking lots of water every day, and regularly exercising could keep your bowel movements regular. Stool softeners might help, too. If you have hemorrhoids, you can talk to your doctor about an ointment or cream that could shrink them.

### What Come Out of Your Body

You have survived your pregnancy this far, and you believe all of those surprises are over. On the day that you have your baby, you are going to be one of the biggest surprises.

During your pregnancy, there is a lot of fluid that your baby has been living inside the amniotic sac. This sac will typically rupture at the onset of labor. This is usually called "your water breaking." Most of the time, the contractions begin before the actual water breaks. There might be times when the doctor will have to break the sac. Like if the woman has been in labor for several hours, the cervix is dilating, but her water hasn't broken.

The amount of water that comes out depends on the term of the baby. If the baby is full-term, there will be about two to three cups. Some women might feel like they need to urinate, which will lead to a gush of fluid as their water breaks. Others might just feel it trickling down their leg due to the baby's head acting as a stopper and keeping the fluid from coming out.

Amniotic fluid is colorless or pale and usually has a sweet smell to it. Your body will replace this fluid every three hours, so you will continue to leak fluid until you deliver your baby.

Other things might be released during labor. Some experience vomiting or nausea, while others could experience diarrhea. Farting is another common occurrence during labor. While you are pushing, you might lose control of your bowels or bladder.

### Joint Mobility

Your body will create the hormone relaxin during pregnancy. This is thought to help get your cervix and pubic area ready for birth. Relaxin will loosen the ligaments in the body. This causes you to be less stable, and you are at a higher risk of injuries. You can easily strain or overstretch yourself, especially at the knees, pelvis, and low back. Any time you are lifting or exercising, take it slow and easy and try not to make any sudden or jerky movements.

### Shoe Size

Although you can't fit into any of the clothes you wore before you got pregnant, you still have all your cute shoes, right? Well, maybe. All of the extra fluid you have right now will cause swollen feet, so you might have to get a bigger shoe. Slip-on shoes tend to be more comfortable, especially when you are pregnant during the hot summer months.

### Nails and Hair

Most women will have changes in their hair growth and texture during pregnancy. Hormones might make your hair grow a lot faster, and you won't have as much fallout. These changes aren't going to be permanent. Most women will lose some hair during their postpartum period or once they stop breast-feeding.

Some women might find they have hair growing in places that they don't want like around their nipples, belly, or face. Changes in the texture of their hair might make it oilier or drier. Some women might even have a slight change to the color of their hair.

Nails can also change during pregnancy. The extra hormones in your body will make the get stronger and grow faster. Some women find that their nails will break and split a lot easier during their pregnancy. Just like the changes to the hair, the changes to their nails won't be permanent, either. If your nails are breaking or splitting easily now, just keep them trimmed short and stay away from the harsh chemicals in nail polish and remover.

### Changes In Skin

Have your friends or family commented that you look like you are glowing? This is just one more effect that hormones can have on your body.

Pregnant women have more blood pumping through their bodies to give more blood to the uterus and other organs like the kidneys. This is going to add more blood to your vessels and will increase oil secretion.

Some women will develop a yellow or brown colored patch of skin on their faces called chloasma or "the mask of pregnancy." Some might see their linea nigra appear down the middle of their stomach. They could have hyperpigmentation of the anal region, external genitalia, and nipples. This just means the skin in these areas has gotten darker.

This hyperpigmentation may not be even so that the darker skin might look like patches of color. Chloasma can't be prevented, but staying away from UV light and wearing sunscreen can lessen its effects.

Acne might appear due to the extra oils in the sebaceous glands. Freckles and moles that you had before you got pregnant might get darker or larger. The majority of these things are going to go away after you give birth.

Some women will get heat rashes due to excessive sweating and dampness. Basically, pregnancy could be an itch time for many women. Your stretching belly can cause flaking and itchy skin. You can ask your doctor for the best creams to help with that. There are many over-the-counter creams that can help or just use some Vitamin E oil.

**Size of Your Bra**

One of the first signs of pregnancy will be an increase in the size of your breasts. Breast growth during the first trimester is caused by high levels of the hormones progesterone and estrogen. The growth during the first trimester might be the end of it, or your breasts might continue to grow during your whole pregnancy.

Your bra size could be affected by your ribcage. While you are pregnant, the capacity of your lungs will increase to allow you to take in more oxygen. This might lead to a larger chest size. You might have to replace your bras throughout your pregnancy.

### Mood Swings

Pregnancy and premenstrual syndrome are alike in several ways. Your hormones will fluctuate, you might feel extremely moody, and your breasts will get larger and be extremely tender. If you were prone to PMS, you would probably have severe mood swings during pregnancy. They could make you cry one minute and be laughing like a hyena the next.

Mood swings are very common. They usually happen during the first trimester and then again at the end of the third trimester.

Some women will get depressed during their pregnancy. If you have any symptoms like mood swings that last more than two weeks, change in your eating habits, and sleep problems, you need to talk to your doctor immediately.

## Problems Concentrating

During your first trimester, morning sickness and being tired all the time can make you feel worn out, and this can cause you to be a bit fuzzy mentally. Even pregnant women who get lots of sleep might have problems concentrating along with periods of being forgetful.

Thinking about your baby can play a role in this, along with hormonal changes. Everything, including doctor's appointments, bills, and work, might not seem as important as the baby and its birth. Coming up with a list is helpful when it comes to remembering all of your important appointments and dates.

## You Want to Nest

Most pregnant women will feel an instinct to nest. This is where you experience a powerful urge to clean or decorate the home in anticipation of your new arrival.

As you get closer to your due date, you might notice that you are washing or cleaning walls, cupboards, or anything that you normally wouldn't even think about doing during your ninth month of pregnancy. This desire to get your home ready is useful; you won't have as many things to do after the baby gets here. Just take it easy and don't overdo it.

Having a birth plan can help tell your doctors about your wishes and how they should handle these aspects of your labor and delivery.

There is a lot of surprises in store for a woman during pregnancy, but none of them are better than how you are going to feel when you hold your newborn baby in your arms for the very first time.

# CONCLUSION

Thank you for making it through to the end of the book; let's hope it was informative and able to provide you with all of the tools you need to know what the pregnancy could be like for you and if you are ready to have a baby.

Pregnancy is an amazing thing for those who long to have a child. It's also a long process that may not go how you may expect it to go.

Everybody's pregnancy is going to look different. There is no set model of how pregnancy is supposed to go or supposed to look like. It's going to affect the woman differently, and there are possible complications. The worst thing you can assume is that you know how your pregnancy is going to work. It's going to only add stress to your already stressed body. Take things in stride. It's the best thing that you can do.

The one fact that remains the same is that pregnancy is an amazing process. It might not be perfect, but most women are in awe of what their body does and how amazing their baby is once they get to hold it.

Deciding whether or not you are ready to have a baby is the most important decision you will have to make. Once you know for certain that you want to have a baby, you can start trying to conceive. And then once you find out you're pregnant, you are at the mercy of your body and the growing child inside of you. Your body knows what to do. There's nothing you will have to really think about. As long as you take care of your body, your body will take care of your baby. Don't worry, though, you'll make it through, as well your baby, and your life will be better than ever.

Finally, if you found this book useful in any way, a review on Amazon is always appreciated!

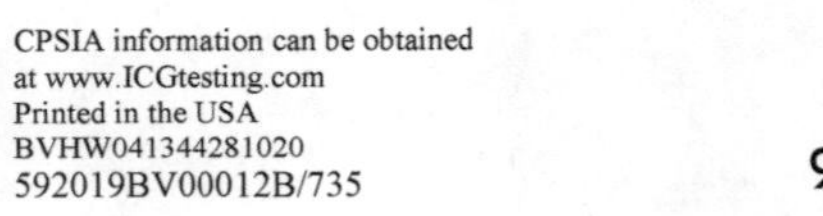

CPSIA information can be obtained
at www.ICGtesting.com
Printed in the USA
BVHW041344281020
592019BV00012B/735

9 781801 131148